Total TORSO Training

GOLD'S GYM® ESSENTIALS

Total TORSO Training

Edward Connors, Peter Grymkowski, Tim Kimber, and Michael J. B. McCormick

CB

CONTEMPORARY BOOKS

Library of Congress Cataloging-in-Publication Data

Total torso training / Edward Connors . . . [et al.] ; with photographs
    by Irvin J. Gelb.
        p.   cm. — (Gold's Gym essentials series ; bk. 2)
    ISBN 0-8092-2788-6
    1. Bodybuilding—Training.   2. Muscle strength.   I. Connors, Ed.
II. Series.
GV546.5.T68   1999
613.7'1—dc21   99-21573
                                                  CIP

Cover design by Todd Petersen
Cover and interior photographs by Irvin J. Gelb
Interior design by Hespenheide Design

Published by Contemporary Books
A division of NTC/Contemporary Publishing Group, Inc.
4255 West Touhy Avenue, Lincolnwood (Chicago), Illinois 60712-1975 U.S.A.
Printed in the United States of America
International Standard Book Number: 0-8092-2788-6
    00 01 02 03 04   VL   15 14 13 12 11 10 9 8 7 6 5 4 3 2

3 4859 00224 2385

CONTENTS

INTRODUCTION

When you saw your first truly huge bodybuilder, what you actually saw was a truly huge torso. Think about it: as humans, we naturally look first at the upper half of the person in front of us. It's only after waking from the initial shock of the cartoonish chest, back, and shoulders of the behemoth that your eyes take note of the arms or legs. Yes, indeed, it was likely the overwhelming size of their torso that made that indelible impression upon your mind, which in turn ignited your bodybuilding passion.

This second book in the Gold's Gym Essentials series presents the actual exercises that have proven to produce the greatest possible increases in lean torso mass in the shortest period of time. We've covered dozens of movements for total development of your back, chest, shoulder traps, and abdominals. You'll find every conceivable approach and angle covered. Barbells, dumbbells, cables, machines, and bodyweight exercises are all described in terms of muscles involved, starting position, and the actual movement itself.

So let's brush up on our bodybuilding basics. In order for you to achieve the maximum results from your training, here are some important basic bodybuilding facts and terms you need to know.

BASIC FACTS AND TERMS

A **repetition** is the completion of both the concentric (positive or lifting motion) and the eccentric (negative or lowering motion) portions of an exercise. For example, in a Barbell Curl, the lifting of the barbell from the front of the thighs to the upper chest is one half of a full repetition. This is known as the **concentric** portion (positive or upward motion) of one repetition in the curl. The final half of a repetition in the Barbell Curl is the lowering of the barbell from the upper chest back to the starting point in front of the thighs. This is called the **eccentric** (negative or lowering motion) of one repetition in the curl.

A **set** is the group of repetitions that is performed without rest, in a back-to-back, nonstop fashion. Again we'll use Barbell Curls as the example. After first warming up sufficiently, your workout calls for, perhaps, 4 sets of Barbell Curls with 90 pounds. Your repetition goal is 10 repetitions for each set. Your first set consists of lifting and lowering the barbell 10 consecutive times. Then the barbell is returned to the floor or rack. You have now completed 1 set of 10 repetitions.

Rest after this first set for a period of 60–120 seconds and then repeat the same process of 10 repetitions with the barbell. You have now completed your second set. This example applies to the majority of bodybuilding exercises with one exception: the type of exercise that calls for each arm or leg to move in an alternating fashion. In these exercises you must perform the movement once for both the right and left sides for it to count as 1 complete repetition.

A **warm-up set** is a set performed with light weights (with little muscular effort) to prepare the muscles for heavier weights.

How long should a workout last? In general, it may take about 50 minutes for an individual to train. On average, for training with one partner, a two to three bodypart workout lasts between 60 and 90 minutes. In actual time spent in the gym, with two people assisting each other, a workout's upper limit timewise is about 75 to 90 minutes. This is with no additional rest other than the two minutes or so between sets and the time it takes to load the weights.

These times do not apply to leg workouts. Due to the tremendous amount of energy and oxygen consumed by the body during leg workouts, in most cases, the legs take the longest time to train correctly. An extreme of 100–150 minutes is not unheard of. More commonly the session will take less than 95 minutes.

TRAINING STRATEGIES

Drop sets are a method of performing your exercise that increases the intensity of your training. In this type of lifting, at the point of momentary muscular failure, the trainer stops the movement long enough to allow your partners to decrease the weight by a certain amount. Your grip and position are maintained while plates are removed or the stack changed. The extended set is then continued till done.

Rest pause sets are similar to drop sets but may be done without the active assistance of partners. At the point of muscular failure, you maintain the grip or position with the resistance load as in drop sets, but the weight remains the same without any adjustment from the spotters at hand. Hands remaining in the training position, you "rest" or "pause" for 15–35 seconds. Then you resume the extended set.

Partial and half repetitions exemplify the principle of overloading in successful bodybuilding. A shortened range of motion allows for heavier than normal weights to be employed. Often partials and half reps are performed using a weight rack or Smith-type machine. Partial reps are the same as half reps but are performed with a higher or lower percentage of completion according to the specified degree of performance. Half reps are reps without the top half of the movement as in curls or without the bottom half as in squats.

An **assisted repetition** is a technique in which, as you fail during the positive or concentric portion of the exercise, your partner(s) helps assist you to complete the full repetition. Correct application of this technique requires experience on the part of your training partners. They must be able to apply just enough help with finishing your rep. If they assist too much, they are doing the work for you.

A **forced repetition** is a similar intensity-increasing technique. The basics are the same as for assisted reps. In forced reps your training partner deliberately applies extra resistance to your reps. The differences between assisted and forced reps are subtle. In assisted reps your partner applies just enough help to finish the repetition. With forced reps the partner applies extra resistance by holding back against the bar or handles. The amount of extra tension placed on the muscle is generally sufficient to see the movement slow just short of actually stopping.

How many days per week should I train? The least number of workouts is 2 days per week. You could set up your training like this:

Day 1: chest, delts, triceps, thighs, and calves
Day 2: back, hamstrings, biceps, abs, and forearms

An example of higher volume training is a 5-days-per-week arrangement. The details of such an approach are:

Day 1: back, traps
Day 2: chest, abs
Day 3: delts, triceps
Day 4: biceps, forearms
Day 5: thighs, calves

Either way you decide to train, it's the recovery after the training that produces growth, not the workouts in isolation. Workouts, food, and recuperation are all integral aspects to successful bodybuilding.

Total sets per body part? The range of 6–14 sets per workout for thighs, back, chest, and delts is appropriate for most bodybuilders. The thighs, chest, back, and delts are considered to be the large muscle groups. Of course you should develop your own numbers that are adjusted according to the number of different muscles being trained that day. The biceps, triceps, calves, forearms, and abs are the smaller muscle groups. For the biceps, triceps, calves, forearms, and abs, a total set range of 3–8 per training session works well.

How many sets per exercise? Take the number of total sets per body part and then divide by the number of exercises. *Example*: Your training routine calls for 6 total sets of biceps exercises. You decide that the two exercises you will use are Barbell Curls and Seated Dumbbell Curls. You would perform 3 working sets (3 sets Barbell Curls and 3 sets Seated Dumbbell Curls) for both exercises after first completing your warm-up sets.

How many repetitions per each set? The range of repetitions per set of an exercise is important. A low repetition count is 5–6 repetitions per set, while a high count would be 12–15 repetitions per set.

With how much weight? As the number of repetitions decreases, you will be using more weight to perform the exercise. Likewise, as you increase the number of repetitions, you'll have to use less weight. In general the biggest bodybuilders used the heaviest weights in their training careers.

Total TORSO Training

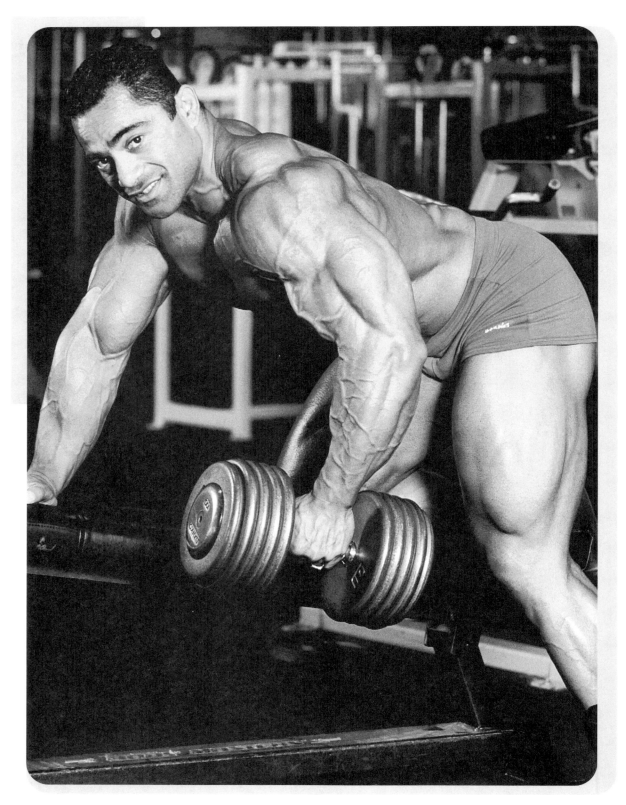

Tevita Aholelei

BACK TRAINING

Of all the body parts, your back is the hardest to hide. Whether your back is wide or narrow will be a matter of choice after reading this chapter. Specifically your "back" is the posterior or dorsal portion of the trunk of your body between your neck and pelvis. The back is divided by a middle furrow that lies over the tips of the spinous processes of the vertebrae.

The back attains muscular perfection when it is both wide and thick. Make no mistake about it, a thick back must be present or the entire torso is compromised in appearance. In order to accomplish the task of developing a radical wingspread, you'll need to use a wide variety of back exercises. Most back movements lend themselves to multiple positions of grip alignment and width.

A key to successful back training is to learn to isolate the pulling motion of your back muscles from the related pulling of your biceps. It takes a good deal of focused concentration to achieve consistent back isolation. For many bodybuilders, the thought of "pulling with your elbows—not with your hands" creates the correct mental image.

The use of lifting straps is another useful option for many bodybuilders. Often the back muscles are considerably stronger than your grip. When this situation occurs, without straps, the set is stopped before the back is thoroughly trained. With appropriate use of straps as needed, the back can be properly attacked from all vital approaches.

This chapter contains complete descriptions of the 22 most effective and productive back exercises ever created. Most, if not all, of these very same movements are observed every day of the week inside Gold's Gym. Success in back development is yours when a thoughtful exercise selection is matched with consistent action.

MUSCLES OF THE BACK

Before we discuss the actual exercises for your back attack, let's get a grip on the anatomical details of the muscles that make up your back. The superficial muscles of the back are large and include the latissimus dorsi, rhomboideus major, and the rhomboideus minor.

The **latissimus dorsi** are large triangular muscles on the thoracic and lumbar areas of the back. The latissimus dorsi extend, adduct, and rotate the arms medially, and draw the shoulders back and down.

The **rhomboideus major** are muscles of the upper back. The rhomboideus major function to draw the scapula toward the vertebral column while supporting it and drawing it slightly upward.

The **rhomboideus minor** are muscles of the upper back lying above and parallel to the rhomboideus major. Their function is the same as for the rhomboideus major.

The deep muscles of the back are the sacrospinalis, teres major and minor, interspinales, intertransversarii, longissimus, multifidi, rotatores, splenius, semispinales, spinales, transversocostal, and transversospinal.

The thick ridges of sinew on either side of the spine are the **sacrospinalis**, also known as the erector spinae. These are the large, fleshy muscles of the back that divide the back into right and left sides. These muscles serve to extend and flex the vertebral column and the head.

The **teres major** are thick, flat muscles arising from the dorsal surface of the scapula. They function to adduct, extend, and rotate the arm medially.

The **teres minor** are cylindrical, elongated muscles also arising from the dorsal surface of the scapula. The teres minor function to rotate the arm laterally and to weakly adduct the arm.

Front Lat Pulldown

Muscles Involved
Front Lat Pulldowns directly stress the latissimus dorsi, serratus anterior, interior intercostal, rhomboideus major and minor, and teres major and minor. Secondary emphasis is placed on the supraspinatus, infraspinatus, posterior deltoid, biceps, brachialis, and the forearm flexor muscles.

Position
Adjust the seat height in front of the weight stack so that your legs are firmly anchored under the pads provided. Now stand up and place your hands with a palms-facing-away-from-you–thumbs-under-the-bar grip.

Your hands should be about shoulder width or slightly wider on the bar. Firmly grasp the bar, straighten your arms, and sit

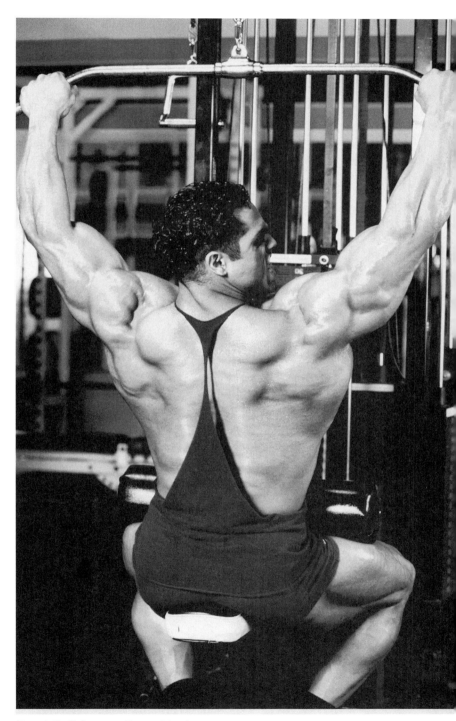

Front Pulldowns Dave Hughes

down while simultaneously locking your legs under the restraining pads. Arch your back and keep it slightly arched during the entire movement.

Movement Performance

Concentrate on pulling your elbows downward and backward as you pull the bar down in front of your neck to touch the upper portion of your chest. Slowly return to the starting position and repeat the movement for the desired rep count.

Tips

If you are strong enough to use a heavier than bodyweight resistance in this movement, then have a spotter assist you into the starting position by pushing firmly down on your shoulders and traps.

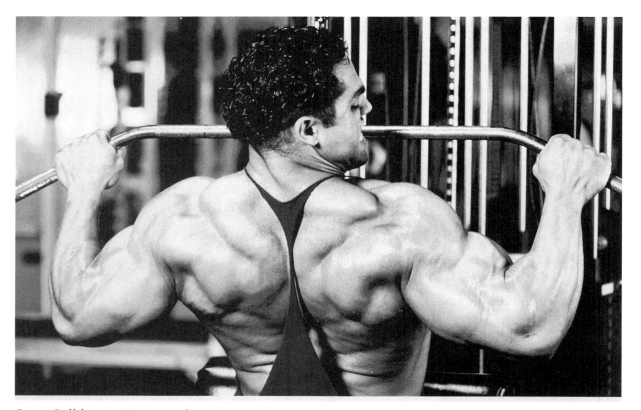

Front Pulldowns Dave Hughes

Changing your grip on the bar will shift the focus of muscular stress when doing pulldowns as follows: wide grip hits more of the upper lat width, while a relatively close grip (4–6 inches) stimulates the lower lat area. Using a pulldown bar with parallel grips will throw additional emphasis onto the middle lat area.

Behind-the-Neck Pulldown

Muscles Involved
Lat pulldowns directly stress the latissimus dorsi, serratus anterior, interior intercostal, rhomboideus major and minor, teres major and minor, supraspinatus, infraspinatus, posterior deltoid, biceps, brachialis, and forearm flexor muscles.

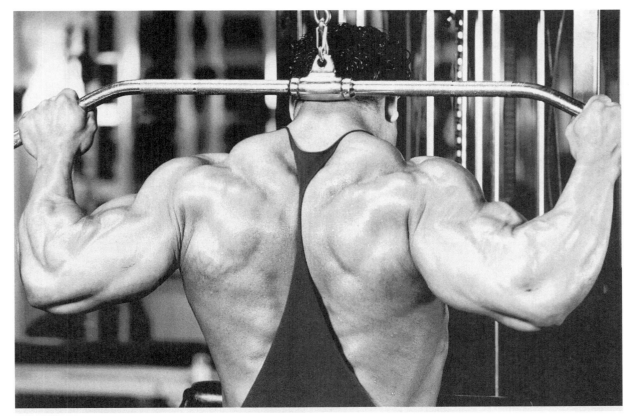

Behind-the-Neck Pulldown Dave Hughes

Position
Adjust the seat height in front of the weight stack so that your legs are firmly anchored under the pads provided. Now stand up and place your hands with a palms-facing-away-from-you–thumbs-under-the-bar grip.

Your hands should be about shoulder width or slightly wider on the bar. Firmly grasp the bar, straighten your arms, and sit down while simultaneously locking your legs under the restraining pads. Lean slightly forward to allow the bar to travel straight down. Keep your back semi-arched during the entire movement.

Movement Performance
Concentrate on pulling your elbows downward and backward as you pull the bar down in back of your neck to a point level with the bottom of your ears. Slowly return to the starting position and repeat the movement for the desired rep count.

Tip
Changing your grip on the bar will shift the focus of muscular stress when doing pulldowns as follows: wide grip hits more of the upper lat width while a shoulder-width (4–6 inches) grip stimulates the lower lat area.

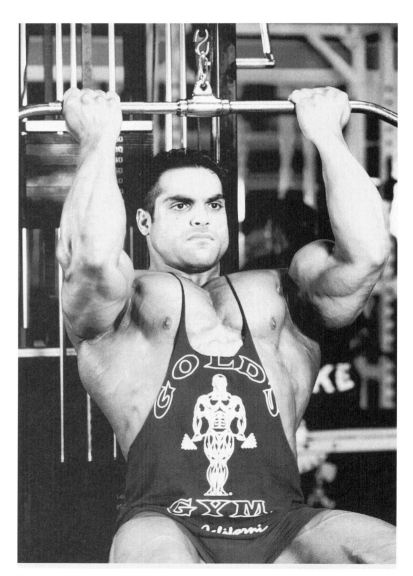

Reverse-Grip Front Pulldown Dave Hughes

Reverse-Grip Front Pulldown

Muscles Involved
Reverse-Grip Front Pulldowns involve the latissimus dorsi, serratus anterior, interior intercostal, and rhomboideus major and minor. A lesser degree of stress is felt by the teres major and minor, supraspinatus, infraspinatus, posterior deltoid, biceps, brachialis, and forearm flexor muscles.

Position
Adjust the seat height in front of the weight stack so that your legs are firmly anchored under the pads provided. Now stand up and place your hands with a palms-facing-away-from-you–thumbs-under-the-bar grip.
    Your hands should be about shoulder width or slightly wider on the bar. Firmly grasp the bar, straighten your arms and sit down while simultaneously locking your legs under the restraining pads. Compared to the conventional pulldowns, your back should be held in a minimal arch.

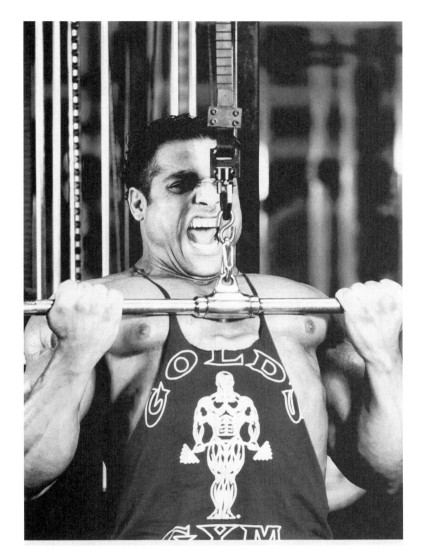

Reverse-Grip Front Pulldown Dave Hughes

Movement Performance
Concentrate on pulling your elbows downward and backward as you pull the bar down in front of your neck to touch the upper

portion of your chest. Slowly return to the starting position and repeat the movement for the desired rep count.

To successfully perform this movement, it is essential that your mental muscle focus is directly on the back muscles. With your hands in a reverse grip there is initially a tendency to involve the biceps too much. This can be avoided by maintaining tension on the back muscles throughout the entire range of motion.

Tip
If you are strong enough to use a heavier than body-weight resistance in this movement, then have a spotter assist you into the starting position by pushing firmly down on your shoulders and traps.

V-Bar Front Pulldown

Muscles Involved
V-Bar Front Pulldowns work the latissimus dorsi, serratus anterior, interior intercostal, rhomboideus major and minor, teres major and minor, supraspinatus, infraspinatus, posterior deltoid, biceps, brachialis, and forearm flexor muscles.

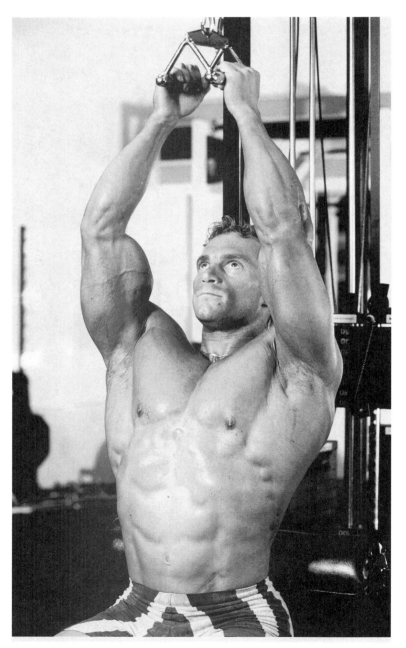

V-Bar Front Pulldown Remi Zuri

Position

Adjust the seat height in front of the weight stack so that your legs are firmly anchored under the pads provided. Now stand up and place your hands with the palms facing together. Your hands should be about 3–4 inches apart.

Straighten your arms and sit down while simultaneously locking your legs under the restraining pads. Arch your back and keep it slightly arched during the entire movement.

Movement Performance

Concentrate on pulling your elbows downward and backward as you pull the bar down in front of your neck to touch the upper portion of your chest. Slowly return to the starting position and repeat the movement for the desired rep count. In this variation of Lat Pulldowns, a phenomenal stretching action is attained.

Tip

This movement developed from bodybuilders performing extreme close-grip chin-ups (or "chins") in which the hands actually touch. The original V-handle chinning bar attachment was widely used at Gold's Gym, Venice, in the '70s.

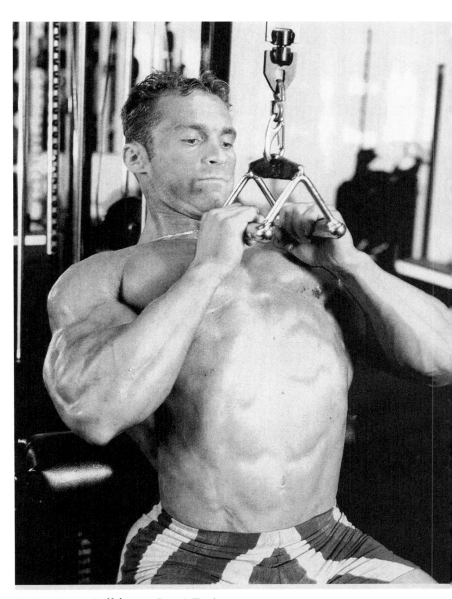

V-Bar Front Pulldown Remi Zuri

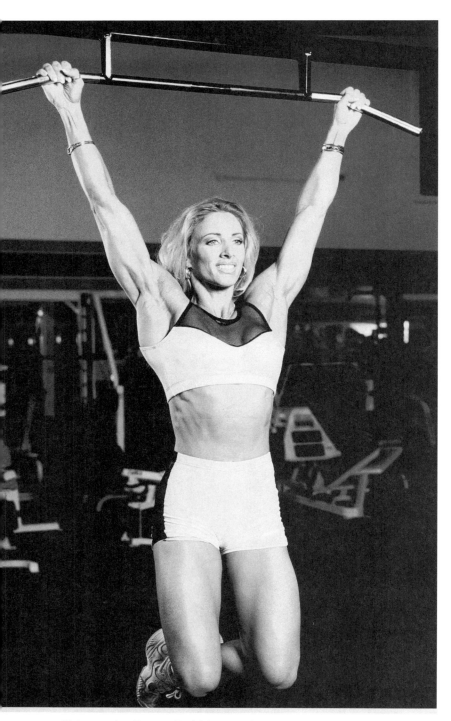

Chin to the Front Debbie Kruck

Chin

Muscles Involved
All varieties of Chins place strong stress on the latissimus dorsi, serratus anterior, interior intercostal, rhomboideus major and minor, teres major and minor, supraspinatus, infraspinatus, posterior deltoid, biceps, brachialis, and forearm flexor muscles.

Position
Depending on your height and the piece of equipment being used, you may need to use a stool or other means of assistance to reach the bar without jumping. Jumping up to grab the chinning bar is risky in terms of injury and is strongly discouraged.

Unless your grip is sufficiently strong, the use of lifting straps is indicated. Often the grip cannot be maintained long enough to allow a full set of 8–12 reps. This is nothing to be discouraged about. As you continue training, your grip will develop along with the rest of your areas of strength.

Wrap your hands around the bar with a thumbs-with-your-palms-facing-away-

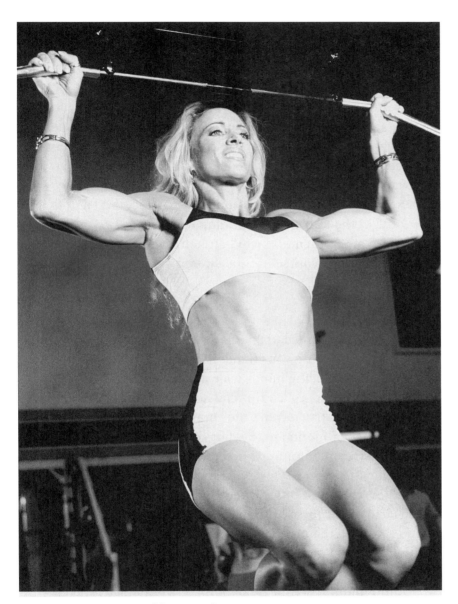

Chin to the Front Debbie Kruck

from-you grip. The width of your grip can be anywhere from 2 inches to a maximum of 36 inches. The closer the grip, the lower on the latissimus dorsi the emphasis. Likewise the wider your grip is, the more you will be stressing your upper lat area. The only restriction is that you must be able to pull your torso up to at least a height of where your chin is above the bar itself.

Movement Performance

Once your grip is firmly set, take your feet off of the stool and allow your arms to reach a full extension. If you are able to simply reach up from a standing position to grab, then draw your lower legs up and behind you to allow the body to hang from the bar.

Now begin to pull yourself up to the correct level and arch your back at the top before beginning to descend. Then reverse the motion and return to the full-stretch starting point. Be careful not to overly relax yourself at the bottom or you could injure your shoulder joints.

Tips

Chins may be performed in a variety of ways according to your training goals. Placing your hands close together targets the lower lats while placing hands wide apart hits the lats higher up. So decide how to approach this classic exercise according to how your physique is structured. Chins may also be performed with a reduced range of motion in the more difficult **Behind-the-Neck Chin**. This style of chinning is reserved for the advanced bodybuilder due to its extraordinary strength requirement.

A **Reverse-Grip Chin** is when you grasp the bar with your palms facing your torso as in Barbell Curls, for example. This allows the biceps a more powerful pulling position. The different position of your hands and arms allows the lats to be blasted in an unusually intense manner.

A minimum repetition goal of 6–8 repetitions with bodyweight is a reasonable gauge to ascertain whether you're in a position to get the full benefit from this exercise. If you're not able to reach that repetition number, perform Pulldowns until you build up the required strength for Chins. If you are gifted or advanced in the number of reps and you're able to grind out more than 12–14 perfect reps, then it's time to start adding extra resistance after your warm-ups are completed.

Additionally, some equipment manufacturers market specifically designed Chin Machines. These chinning machines provide
a counterbalanced platform to stand or kneel on that acts as a
spotter would to assist in the process of raising your chin to the
level of the bar.

Straight-Arm Pulldown

Muscles Involved
Straight-Arm Pulldowns
stress the latissimus dorsi, serratus anterior, interior intercostal, rhomboideus major
and minor, teres major and
minor, and infraspinatus muscles. An increased shift
toward stressing the smaller
non-latissimus muscles occurs
during this movement.

Position
Stand in front of an overhead
cable pulley or pulldown
machine. Using a straight bar
attached to the cable, place
your hands about shoulder
width apart. Take a step or
two back in order to place
your upper body in a moder-
ate forward tilt with your
lower body perpendicular to
the floor.

A visual cue to the cor-
rect starting position is to pic-
ture a clock at 6:05. Your
lower body is to be in the hour

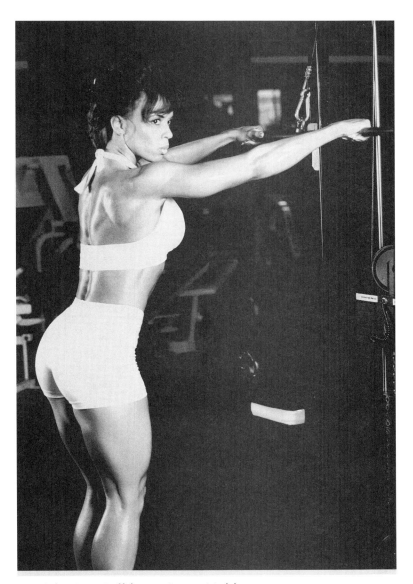

Straight-Arm Pulldown Saryn Muldrow

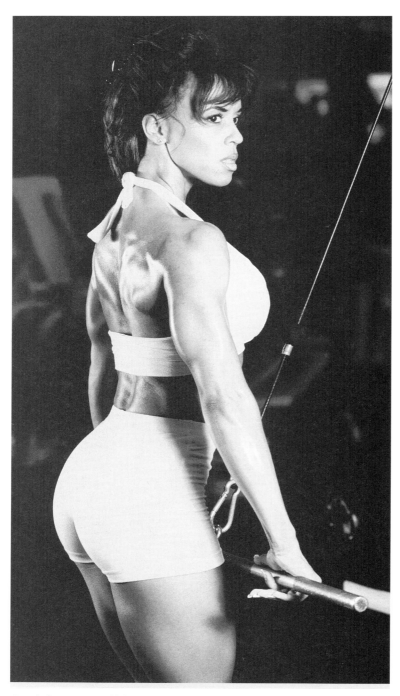

Straight-Arm Pulldown Saryn Muldrow

hand alignment with your upper body as the minute hand. This exercise does not require heavy weights to be used. Perhaps start with 30–40 percent of the weight used for Front Pulldowns.

Movement Performance
With your arms straight, push your hands down toward the top of your thighs. This exercise requires you to focus your energy through your hands as opposed to conventional pulldowns in which you concentrate on pulling with the elbows. Attempt to feel your back muscles tightly spreading as you reach near midpoint in the movement.

As the bar makes contact with your thighs, reverse the direction of the movement and return to the top position. Hold the tension in your back muscles during the return to starting position.

Tip
Moving the grip inside so that the hands are 2–3 inches apart increases the workload for the serratus anterior and internal intercostal muscles.

One-Arm Seated Low Cable Row

Muscles Involved

This movement is for developing all of the back muscles: trapezius, latissimus dorsi, serratus anterior, interior intercostal, rhomboideus major and minor, teres major and minor, supraspinatus,
infraspinatus, posterior deltoid, and erector spinae. Strong stress
is also placed upon the posterior deltoid, biceps, brachialis, and
forearm flexor muscles.

Position

Bend forward and grasp the handle. Place your feet against the
foot bars at the front end of the apparatus seat, straighten your

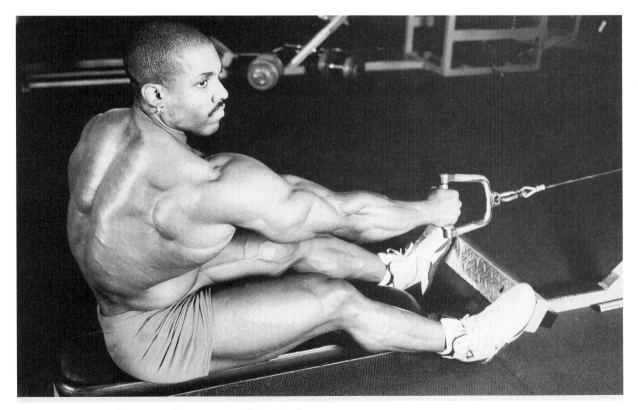

One-Arm Seated Low Cable Row Melvin Anthony

arms, and sit down on the seat, keeping your knees slightly bent throughout the entire movement. Place your non-lifting hand against the knee on the same side. Your torso will be twisted from your waist to your shoulder on the side being trained.

Movement Performance
Sit back to a point just beyond perpendicular to the floor while at the same time you pull the handle back and in toward your belt. Try to touch the handle to the top of your illius (hip bone). Reverse the movement, and while maintaining constant tension, allow the handle to return to the original position.

Tip
Twisting the handle as you pull toward your waist to the right or left of the original position will optimize the isolation between back muscles.

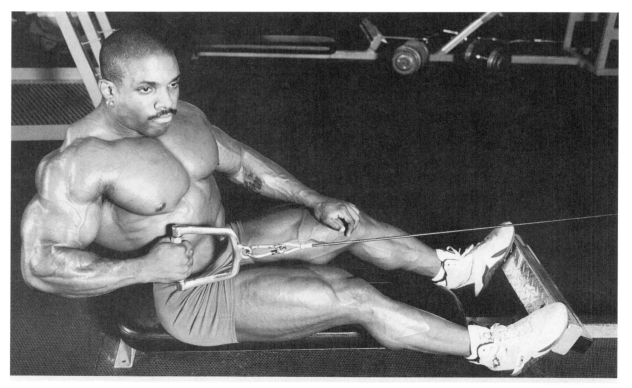

One-Arm Seated Low Cable Row Melvin Anthony

V-Bar Seated Low Cable Row

Muscles Involved

This is an excellent movement for developing all of the back muscles: trapezius, latissimus dorsi, serratus anterior, interior intercostal, rhomboideus major and minor, teres major and minor, supraspinatus, infraspinatus, posterior deltoid, and erector spinae. Stress is also placed upon the posterior deltoid, biceps, brachialis, and forearm flexor muscles.

Position

Most commonly this movement is performed with a v-shaped handle that allows you to take a narrow grip with your palms facing inward toward each other. The handle may also be straight.

Grasp the handle or bar. Place your feet against the foot bars at the front end of the apparatus seat, straighten your arms, and sit down on the seat, keeping your knees slightly bent throughout the entire movement. Sit upright at a 90-degree angle to the floor. Remember to always wear your lifting belt and to maintain an arched back.

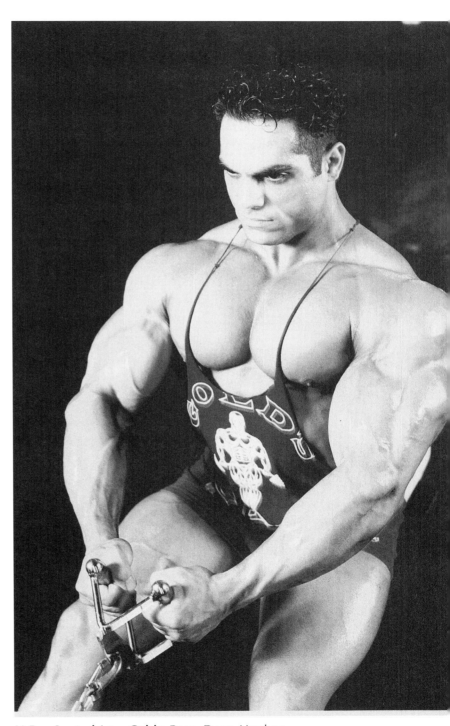

V-Bar Seated Low Cable Row Dave Hughes

Movement Performance

Keeping your elbows in tight against your sides, pull the handle back toward your lifting-belt buckle. Once the handle touches the buckle, squeeze the upper back together and slowly, under control, lower the weight back to the starting point.

Various opinions exist as to how far forward, if at all, you should lean toward the weight stack. The best advice is to avoid any excess bending of the waist when performing Seated Pulley Rows.

It stands to reason that you are attempting to build the thickness in the latissimus dorsi area and are not attempting to perform a modified Deadlift. In general, don't lean forward past a point slightly beyond 90 degrees. There is no chance of mistaking the stretch placed on your upper- and mid-back areas when this exercise is performed correctly as indicated.

Tips

This movement is most frequently performed from a low pulley machine, but it can also be performed from a high pulley set 3–5 feet above the floor. There are also several types of handles that can be used, the most common of which is a V-shaped handle that can position the palms facing together about 6–8 inches apart.

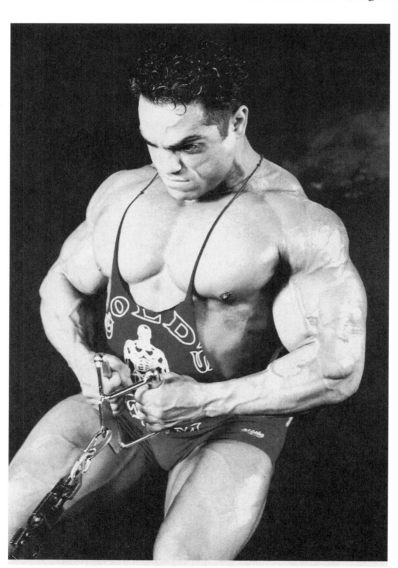

V-Bar Seated Low Cable Row Dave Hughes

Using a straight bar 2–3 feet long will allow you to use a thumbs-over or thumbs-under grip of many different widths. Finally there are arrangements in which two handles are connected together by a cable, which is then attached to the pulley cable itself.

Reverse-Grip Seated Low Cable Row

Muscles Involved
This is an excellent movement for developing all of the same back muscles as the One-Arm and V-Bar Low Cable Rows.

Position
The handle used is straight. Take hold of the handle with a slightly narrower than shoulder width grip, palms facing up (as in Barbell Curls). Your feet are placed against the foot bars at the front end of the apparatus seat. Sit down on the seat, keeping your knees slightly bent during the movement. Sit upright at a 90-degree angle to the floor.

Movement Performance
Keeping your elbows in tight against your sides, pull the handle back toward your lifting-belt buckle. Once the handle touches the buckle, squeeze the upper back together and slowly, under control, lower the weight back to the starting point.

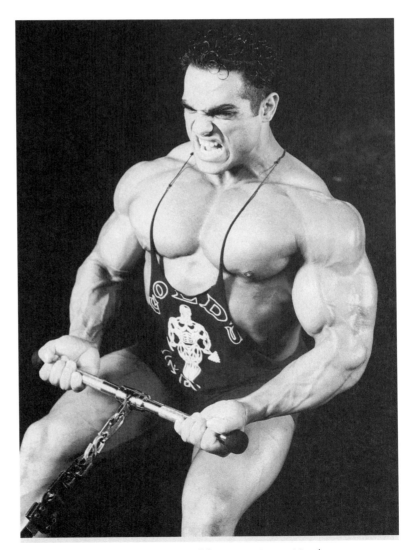

Reverse-Grip Seated Low Cable Row Dave Hughes

One-Arm Dumbbell Bent-Over Row

Muscles Involved

As in the previous movements, One-Arm Dumbbell Bent-Over Rows are a complete back exercise that hits the trapezius, latissimus dorsi, serratus anterior, interior intercostal, rhomboideus major and minor, teres major and minor, supraspinatus, infraspinatus, and posterior deltoid muscles. Due to the angles of muscular motion involved, One-Arm Dumbbell Bent-Over Rows heavily recruit the action of the erector spinae, though not as much as other bent-over movements. Stress is also placed upon the posterior deltoid, biceps, brachialis, and forearm flexor muscles.

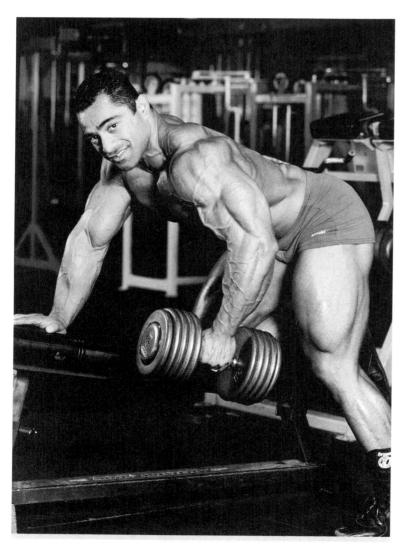

One-Arm Dumbbell Bent-Over Row Tevita Aholelei

Position

Place a dumbbell at one side of a flat bench. Kneel with your right knee and lower leg on the bench and place your right hand about 2 feet ahead of your right knee.

Reach down and grab the dumbbell with your left hand. Completely straighten your left arm and slightly rotate your left shoulder downward to fully stretch your left lat muscle group.

Movement Performance
Keeping your elbow in close to your side, slowly pull the dumbbell directly upward and roll your left delt area as the dumbbell touches the edge of your lower ribs. Lower the weight back into the bottom position and repeat for the desired rep count.

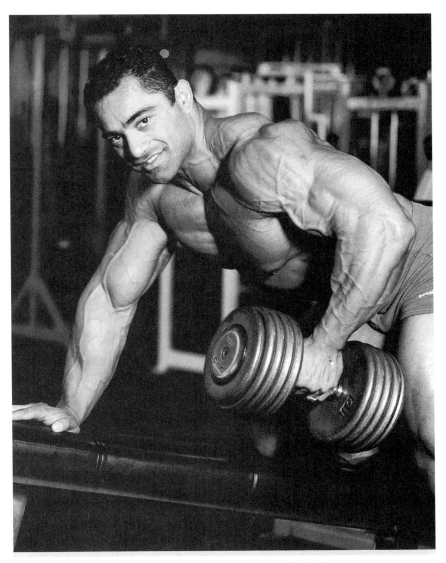

One-Arm Dumbbell Bent-Over Row Tevita Aholelei

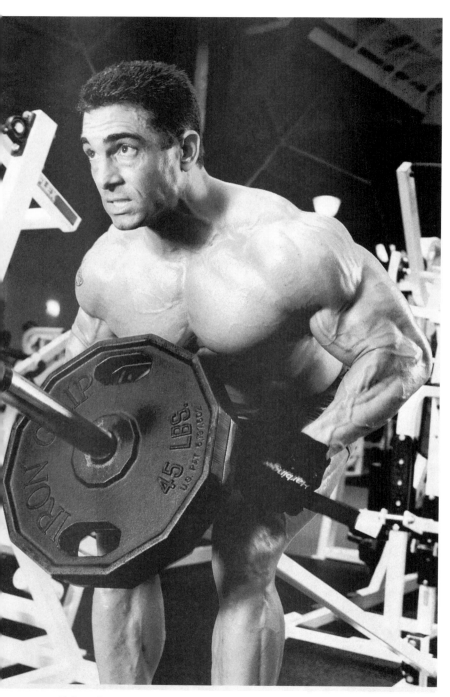

T-Bar Bent-Over Row Kostandinos Malliarodas

T-Bar Bent-Over Row

Muscles Involved
T-Bar Bent-Over Rows launch
an assault upon your trapezius, latissimus dorsi, serratus
anterior, interior intercostal,
rhomboideus major and
minor, teres major and minor,
supraspinatus, infraspinatus,
and posterior deltoid muscles.

Position
Load the apparatus and place
your feet on the platform
behind the handles. Bend over
at the waist with a strong
arch to the lower back.
Remember to use your belt for
this movement.
    Grab the handles and
straighten your legs just short
of completely locking them
out, leaving a slight bend at
the knees. This will raise the
bar from its resting point and
bring your torso to slightly
above parallel.

Movement Performance
Slowly pull the weight
upward, keeping your elbows
tight against your sides, until
it touches your chest. Draw
the shoulders together at the
top of the movement for an

intense contraction. Slowly reverse the movement and lower yourself into the bottom starting position. Repeat until the desired number of reps are completed.

Tip
Various grips can be used for this movement: straight, close, shoulder-width, and V-bar.

Machine T-Bar Bent-Over Row

Muscles Involved
Major emphasis is placed on the target muscles: the latissimus dorsi, serratus anterior, interior intercostal, rhomboideus major and minor, teres major and minor, supraspinatus, and infraspinatus. Significant work is performed by the biceps, brachialis, and forearm flexor muscles. Secondary stress is placed upon the trapezius and posterior deltoids. The muscles of the erector spinae are not significantly worked by the movement.

Position
Lie chest down, resting on the pads as provided, and grasp the handles firmly. Make sure that your lower body is securely positioned.

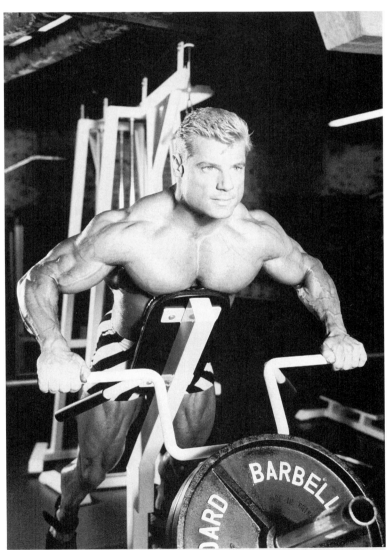

Machine T-Bar Bent-Over Row Joe Lazarro

Movement Performance

Release the weight by raising the handles or bar upward to begin the movement. Slowly lower the weight to the point of full extension. From this point pull the weight upward until you have reached the fullest possible degree of muscular contraction and squeeze the muscle of your upper back. Reverse the movement with a controlled lowering and repeat the sequence for the desired number of reps.

Tip

Most machines allow for a variety of hand placement widths in order to allow for a total back attack, so find the best for your physique and begin the blasting process.

One-Arm Seated Hammer Row/
Two-Arm Alternating Seated Hammer Row

Muscles Involved

In this particular movement, the manufacturers have done an outstanding job of designing highly effective equipment in a wide variety of styles. Common to all of these great designs is tremendous isolation of the latissimus dorsi, serratus anterior, interior intercostal, rhomboideus major and minor, teres major and minor, supraspinatus, and infraspinatus muscles. Significant work is performed by the biceps, brachialis, and forearm flexor muscles. Due to the efficiency of design, the erector spinae muscles have been largely isolated out of the movement.

Position

Assume a position on the machine's seat facing the upright padded area. Adjust the seat for your height so that when your arms are extended straight in front of you, they are in line with the gripping area on the equipment.

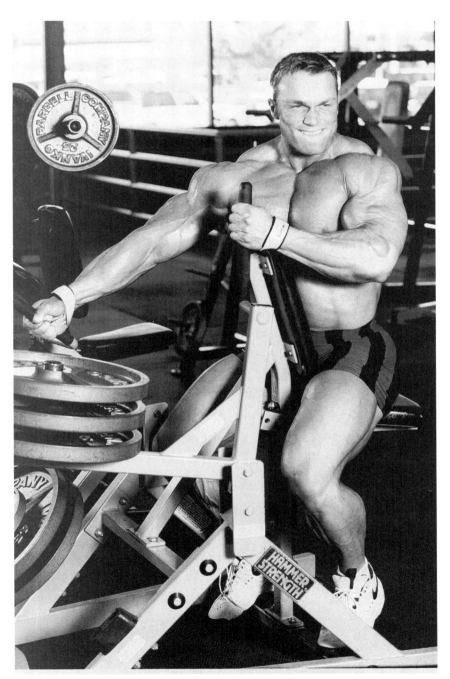

One-Arm Seated Hammer Row Erik Fromm

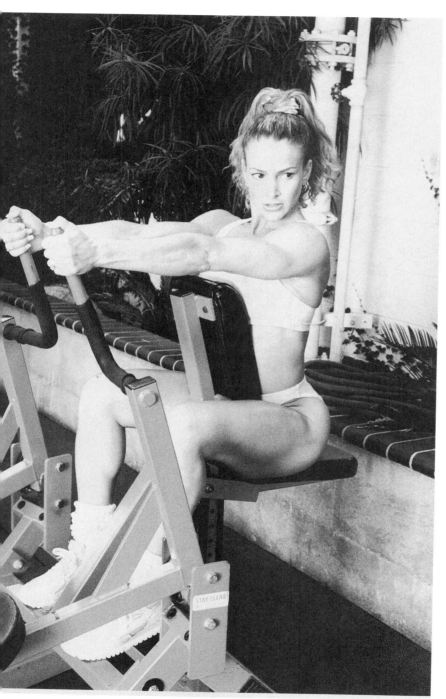

Two-Arm Alternating Seated Hammer Row Mia Finnegan

Position your feet firmly and lean forward so that your chest is touching the upright pads. Grasp the handles firmly and sit erect by leaning slightly back in order to engage the machine's resistance. Position your feet as appropriate for height and equipment.

Movement Performance
Keeping your elbows just below shoulder level, slowly pull your right elbow as far back as is comfortable while maintaining the starting position with your left arm. Reverse the movement to lower the weight back into the starting position. Repeat the sequence for the left side. Upon completing the left arm you have performed one repetition. Continue for the desired number of reps.

Two-Arm Dumbbell Bent-Over Row

Muscles Involved
Performing Bent-Over Rows with two dumbbells instead of one barbell allows you more freedom of movement with your hands. This exercise is

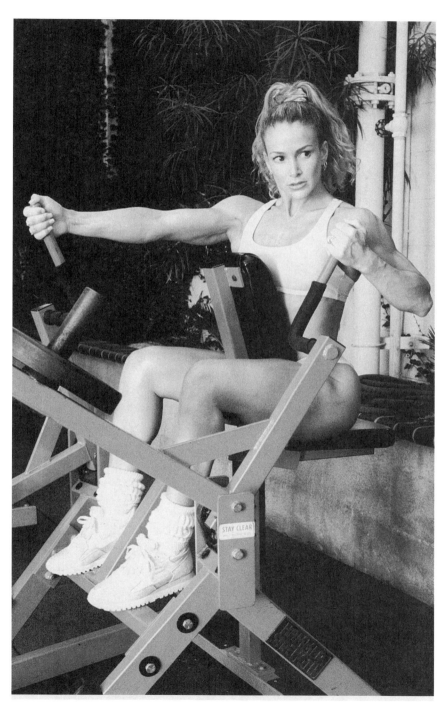

Two-Arm Alternating Seated Hammer Row Mia Finnegan

not performed widely because it is difficult to perform correctly. It does place significant workload on your trapezius, latissimus dorsi, serratus anterior, interior intercostal, rhomboideus major and minor, teres major and minor, supraspinatus, infra-spinatus, and posterior deltoid muscles.

Due to the angles of muscular motion involved, Two-Arm Dumbbell Bent-Over Rows intensely involve the erector spinae to a much greater degree than do rowing movements that are designed with your torso supported. Stress is also placed upon the posterior deltoid, biceps, brachialis, and forearm flexor muscles.

Position
Choose two dumbbells, place them on the floor in front of you, and stand with your toes about shoulder-width apart and angled slightly outward. Unlock your legs throughout the entire movement, and as in all types of rowing move-ments, keep your lower back in an arched position.

Movement Performance
Keeping your elbows close to your sides, slowly pull the dumbbells directly backward until they touch your lower

Two-Arm Dumbbell Bent-Over Row Dave Hughes

rib cage area. Lower them back into the starting position and repeat for the desired rep count.

Tips
You can perform this movement with your palms facing the legs, or facing toward each other.

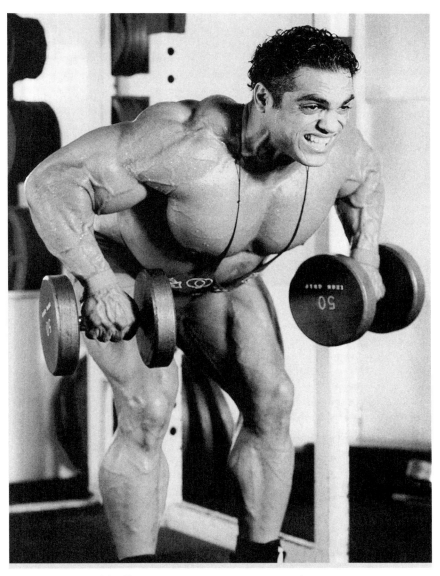

Two-Arm Dumbbell Bent-Over Row Dave Hughes

Barbell Bent-Over Row

Muscles Involved

This is an excellent—maybe even the best—back thickness movement known to man. The stress is on your trapezius, latissimus dorsi, serratus anterior, interior intercostal, rhomboideus major and minor, teres major and minor, supraspinatus, infraspinatus, posterior deltoid, erector spinae, biceps, brachialis, and forearm flexor muscles.

As you perhaps know, all rowing-type back movements emphasize thickness, while in a general sense, the pulldown- and chinning-type moves are associated with increased width.

Position

It is essential to wear a lifting belt and to keep your lower back tightly arched throughout the entire range of sets from the first warm-up to your heaviest stack of plates. Straps are useful if a strong grip has not yet been developed. Stand about 1 1/2 feet back from a bar that, when loaded with a 45-lb. plate on each side, rests near the midpoint of your shin.

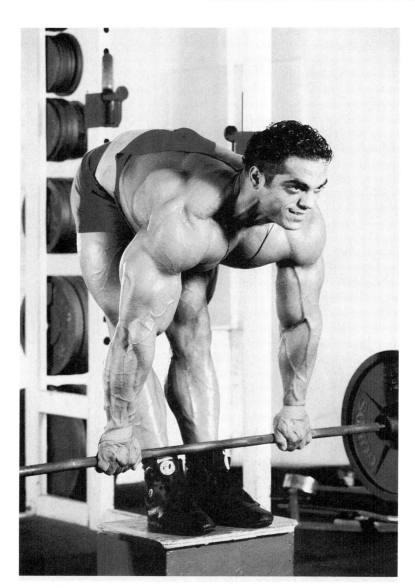

Barbell Bent-Over Row Dave Hughes

Squat down and grasp the bar with a shoulder-width thumbs-over grip. Keeping the arch in your lower back, straighten your legs just short of locking your knees. Your upper body will be just above the bar and parallel to the floor. This will bring your bar to a point at which the plates clear the floor so that you will not be able to rest the bar at the bottom position. Your legs should be just slightly bent at the knees.

Movement Performance
Moving only your arms, slowly pull the bar back at a slight angle so that it touches the buckle on your belt. As you pull the bar toward the buckle, your upper arms should travel out away from your torso at 45-degree angles. As the bar touches the buckle, begin to lower it back to the starting position without exaggerating the stretch by allowing the lower back to move from its starting point.

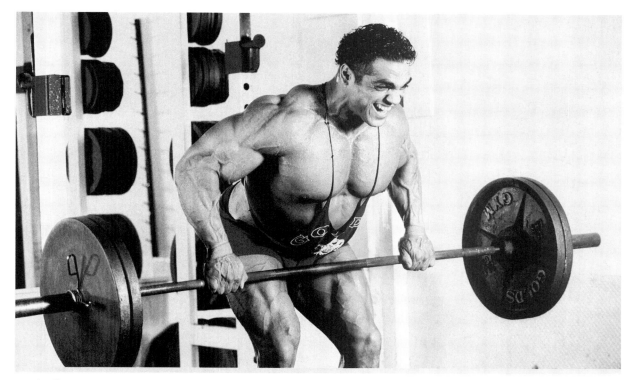

Barbell Bent-Over Row Dave Hughes

In other words, at no time during the movement should you bend at the waist. By maintaining your back in an arched position and not allowing the waist to bend, you will keep the stress on the lats and off the lower back! As you reach the starting position, attempt to feel your lats being stretched. Repeat the movement for the desired number of reps.

Tips
You can use a variety of grip widths as you perform your Bent-Over Rows. Your grip can be as close as having your thumbs touching each other in the center of the bar or as far as a collar-to-collar width. For anyone with a lower back injury, you may utilize a bench at the correct height to rest your head against for additional support.

Reverse-Grip Barbell Bent-Over Row

Muscles Involved
Here the recruitment of muscle groups is the same as for regular Barbell Bent-Over Rows except that many champion bodybuilders feel that more stress is allocated for the lower portion of your latissimus.

Position
With either a straight barbell or an EZ Curl bar, assume the same starting position as for regular Bent-Over Rows except reverse your grip so that your palms are facing away from your shins. Straighten your legs to a point where your torso is slightly above a 45-degree angle to the floor. Bend your knees more than you do for a regular Bent-Over Barbell Row.

Movement Performance
You will repeat the same execution of the movement as in conventional Bent-Over Rows with the following differences:

- Your elbows are actually drawn back at an angle toward your waist as opposed to straight up and down because of the increased bend in your knees.

- Lower the bar back to the starting point using a slower negative or eccentric motion. (You are in a structurally advantageous position because of the elevation of your upper body beyond parallel.)

Caution

Be aware that the ability of the back to handle massive poundages can quickly overwhelm the lifting capacity of the biceps, resulting in muscle tears.

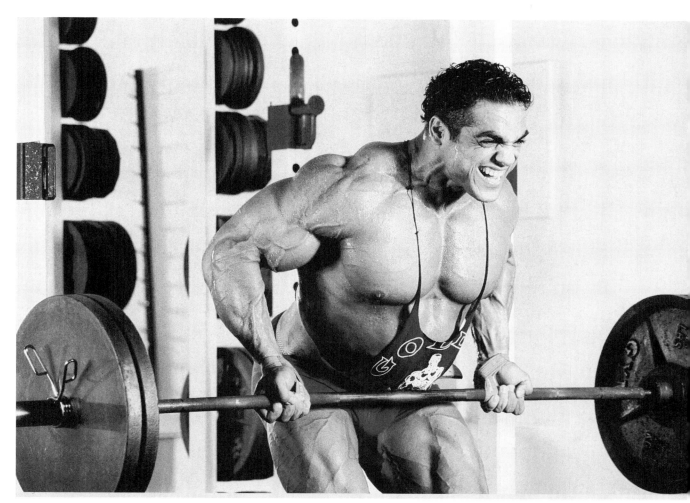

Reverse-Grip Barbell Bent-Over Row Dave Hughes

Dumbbell-Across-Bench Pullover

Muscles Involved
The areas of stress are the latissimus dorsi, pectorals, triceps, serratus anterior, interior intercostal, rhomboideus major and minor, teres major and minor, supraspinatus, infraspinatus, and posterior deltoid muscles.

Position
Lie across the center of a flat bench in a perpendicular, or "T," position. Your upper back and rear delts should be the point of contact with the bench, with your head well off the bench and feet lower than your hips.

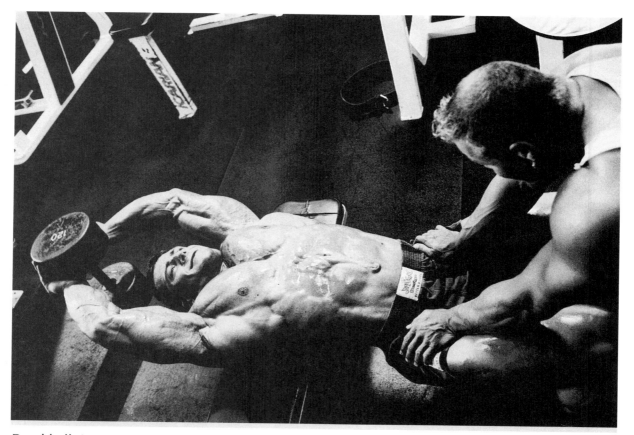

Dumbbell-Across-Bench Pullover Jean-Pierre Fux

Place your hands under the plates of the dumbbell so that your thumbs are around the handle and your fingers are locked together and flat against the plates.

Movement Performance

From a point above your fore-head, slowly lower the dumb-bell to just off the floor. This is an extreme stretch so be careful not to lower the weight quickly. Maintain the feet at a lower point than your hips without allowing the hips to rise more than 1–2 inches as you perform the exercise. Hold the bottom position for a split second and then slowly return to the top position and repeat for the desired number of reps.

Machine Pullover

Muscles Involved

This exercise has been called the squat of upper body movements because of its phenomenal degree of total upper torso stress. As with the other types of pullovers, the stress is on the latissimus dorsi and pectorals; slightly less stress is on the triceps, serratus anterior, interior intercostal, rhomboideus major and minor, teres major and minor, supraspinatus, infraspinatus, and posterior deltoid muscles.

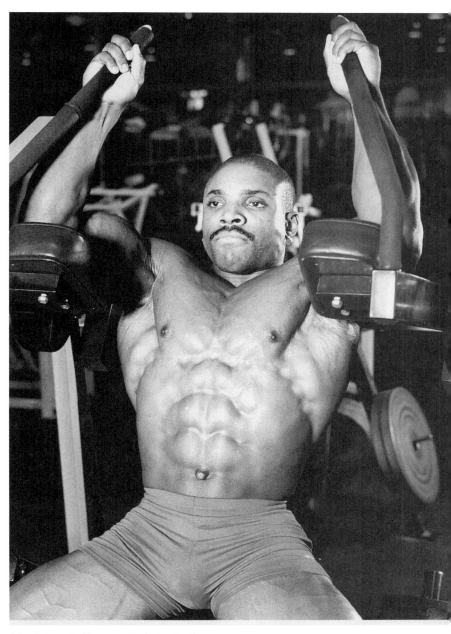

Machine Pullover Melvin Anthony

The benefit from a Machine Pullover is that the lats are isolated to a very high degree because pushing with your elbows removes the biceps involvement. The biceps are weak when compared to the power of your lats.

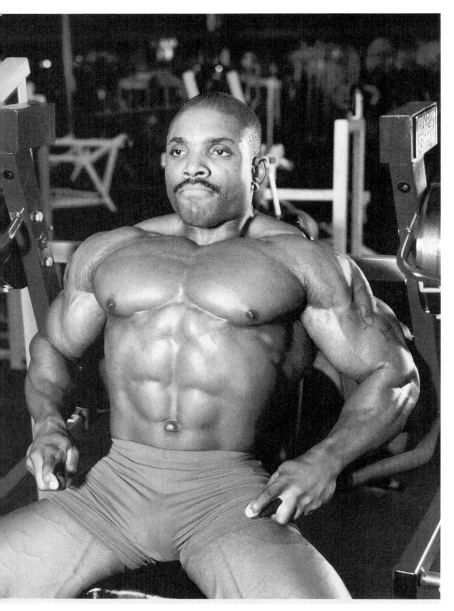

Machine Pullover Melvin Anthony

Position

The correct performance of this movement is similar among the various manufacturers and their respective machines. The key element is to position yourself on the seat so that when your arms are in the overhead position your shoulder joints are in line with the machine's center point or axis of rotation.

Be sure to use the equipment's seat belt or other means of restraint if one is provided. Foot pads are generally provided to allow the arm/elbow pads to be brought to a starting position without assistance. Place the elbows against the pads and take a relaxed grip on the area for your hands.

It is important to make every attempt to isolate the motion so that the elbows are the point of contact with the machine. In an ideal setting the hands would not even need to be involved. This type of focus leads to tremendous isolation of the lats. The more you can perform this exercise focusing on driving with the elbows through the entire range of motion, the better for ultimate back growth.

Slowly release the foot pedal or bar and allow the elbows to be drawn upward above and slightly behind your head. A definite stretch is required to gain maximum benefit from the movement. However, do not allow the machine's resistance to overwhelm your degree of flexibility.

Movement Performance

With your elbows pushing against the pads, bring the elbows down and in front of your torso as far as possible. Do not use your hands to pull on the bar or handles. Bring the elbows to just beyond the plane of your back. Hold the bottom position for a 1–2 second count to obtain a peak contraction. Slowly return to the starting point and repeat for the desired number of reps.

Barbell Pullover (Bent-Arm Pullover)

Muscles Involved

This free-weight movement launches an assault against the latissimus dorsi, pectorals, triceps, biceps, serratus anterior, interior intercostal, rhomboideus major and minor, teres major and minor, supraspinatus, infraspinatus, and posterior deltoid muscles.

Position

Take a thumb-over-bar grip on a barbell with about 6 inches between your hands. Be careful to use collars if the bar is not permanently set. Lie flat on a flat bench with your head off one end and your feet securely positioned at the other end. Rest the bar across your chest with your elbows bent at your sides.

Movement Performance

Keeping your arms bent and your elbows as close together as possible, slowly bring the barbell up in an arch across your face and down behind your head to a point just above the floor. Always maintain control during this exercise, especially during the lowering. Pull the bar up and reverse the same path to where the bar once again rests across your chest. Repeat for the desired number of reps.

Hyperextension

Muscles Involved
This excellent movement effectively isolates the erector spinae, gluteus (maximus, minimus, and medius), biceps femoris (hamstring), senitendinosus, semimembranosus, gracilis, and adductor magnus muscles.

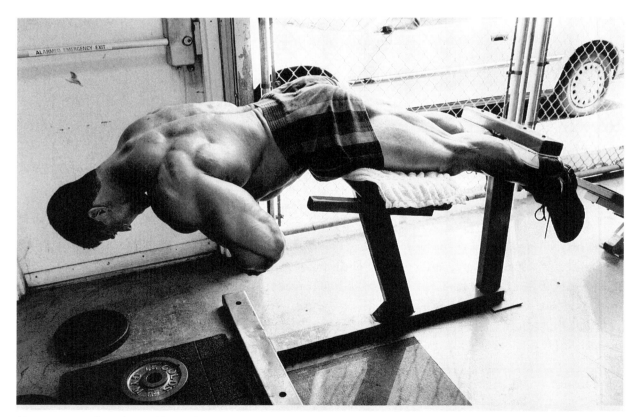

Hyperextension Jean-Pierre Fux

Position

Usually, this exercise is performed on a special bench constructed specifically for it. Stand facing the larger pad. Lean forward and grasp the handles in front of the pad to lever your body into position. Your hips should be across the larger pads with the backs of your ankles resting beneath the smaller pads at the back of the apparatus. Be sure to hold your legs straight throughout the movement. Your arms are to be clasped loosely in back of your head or folded across the top of your chest. The starting position is with your upper body hanging with your head a couple of inches from the floor.

Movement Performance

Arch upward and backward until you rise above the point of being parallel to the floor. Excessive arching of the back is not only ineffective but also is injurious. Return to the original starting point (without rounding your back and losing any of the arch) and repeat the movement for the desired number of reps.

Tips

Resistance can be added to this exercise by holding a light

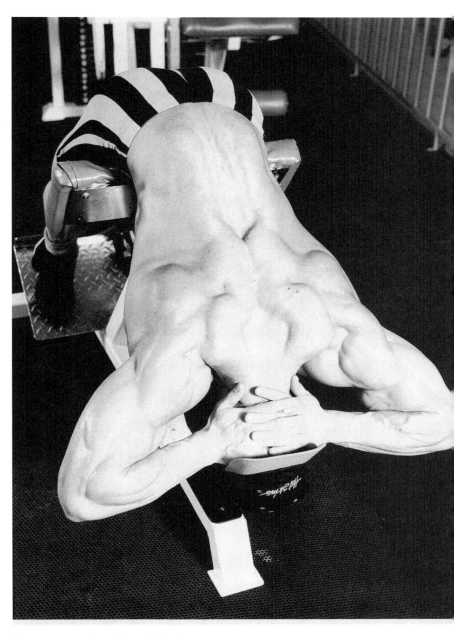

Hyperextension Remi Zuri

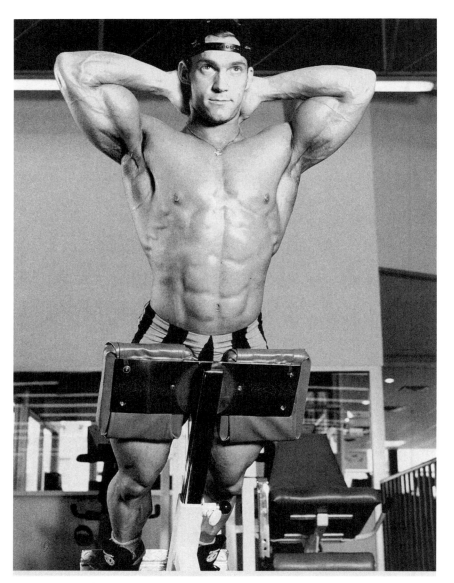

Hyperextension Remi Zuri

barbell or loose barbell plate against the back of your head and neck. If you do not have access to a hyperextension bench for this exercise, you can still do the movement. Rest across a very sturdy, high table or exercise bench. Have a training partner either sit or lie across your legs to hold you in place.

Stiff-Leg Deadlift

Muscles Involved

This movement marshals the muscles of your erector spinae, gluteus (maximus, minimus, and medius), biceps femoris (hamstring),
senitendinosus, semimembranosus, gracilis, and adductor magnus
muscles. Secondary emphasis is on your upper back muscles.

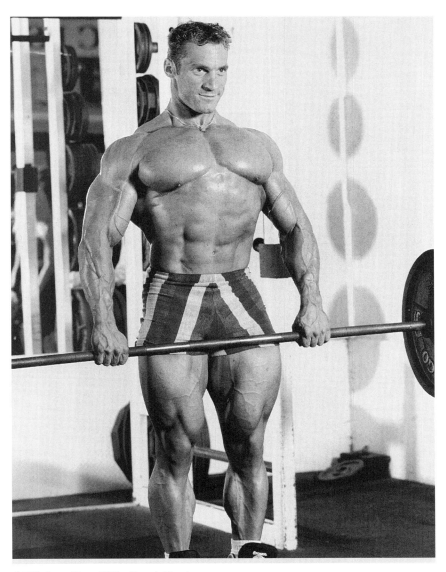

Stiff-Leg Deadlift Remi Zuri

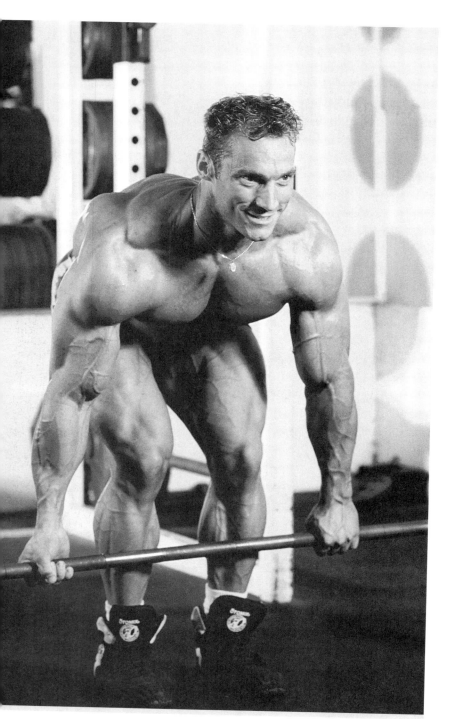

Stiff-Leg Deadlift Remi Zuri

Position
The old practice of standing on a bench to perform this movement has gone out of favor over the last few years. When performed correctly, there is no need for an exaggerated stretching of the hands past the tops of your socks. Take a shoulder-width over-grip on the barbell and stand erect with it, keeping your arms straight and resting the barbell across your upper thighs.

Movement Performance
Maintain a slight bend at the knee the entire time. With your lower back arched, bend forward at the waist and lower the bar downward until the plates just touch the floor, do not rest, and reverse the direction of the bar until you once again stand erect. Repeat the move for the desired number of repetitions.

Tip
Two dumbbells may be used in place of a single barbell.

Good Morning

Comments
When performing this exercise, keep the weight light.

Muscles Involved

This exercise directly stresses the erector spinae, gluteus (maximus, minimus, and medius), biceps femoris (hamstring), senitendinosus, semimembranosus, gracilis, and adductor magnus muscles. Modest secondary stress is placed on your upper back.

Position

Lift a very light barbell to a position across your shoulders and behind your head. Balance the bar in this position during the movement. Remember the bar will try to slide down over your head, so hold on firmly! Place your feet about shoulder-width apart and point your toes directly forward. Stand erect with your knees in a slightly bent position.

Movement Performance

Slowly bend forward at the waist, keeping your back firmly arched the entire time. As soon as your torso has descended past the point of being parallel to the floor, reverse the movement and raise yourself back to a standing position. Repeat the exercise for the desired number of repetitions.

Tip

A workout belt should be worn during this exercise.

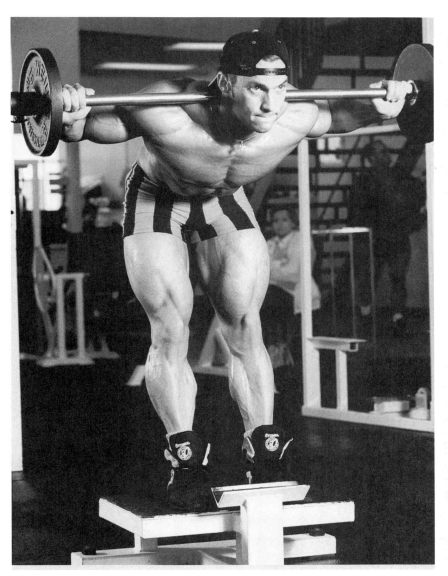

Good Morning Remi Zuri

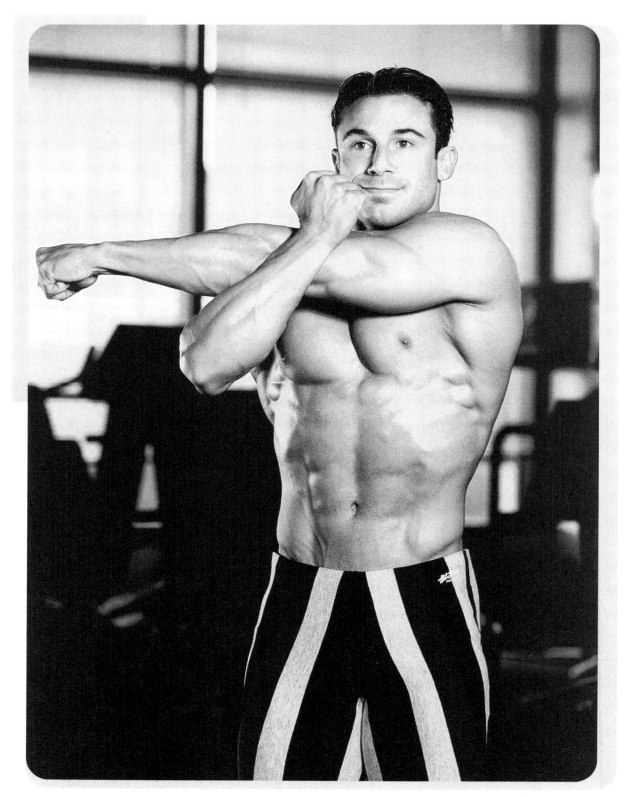

Shoulder Stretch Erik Kaufmann

2
SHOULDER AND TRAPEZIUS TRAINING

Tailors add pads to jackets in order to create the appearance of shoulder width and size. Bodybuilders have done much the same thing for years but with weights, not fabric. Building a set of cannonball shaped deltoids is one of the best strategies for the creation of visual width.

Even though in terms of muscle volume the deltoids are relatively small, the muscles of your shoulders, or the deltoid group, are among the most visually impressive body parts. Melon-size shoulders are impossible to conceal; they mark you as a successful bodybuilder.

MUSCLES OF THE SHOULDER AND TRAPEZIUS

The **deltoid** muscles are large, thick triangular muscles that cover the shoulder joints. The deltoids serve to abduct, flex, extend, and rotate the arms. They arise from various surfaces of the clavicle, acromion, and scapula, and they insert, with a thick tendon, into the humerus. The deltoids are also known as the deltoideis.

The **trapezius** is a large, flat triangular muscle of the shoulder and upper back. It acts to rotate the scapula, raise the shoulder, and abduct and flex the arm.

The following muscles are all involved in moving a shoulder joint:

- Deltoid—abducts, flexes, extends, and rotates the arm
- Trapezius—raises the shoulder, abducts and flexes the arm
- Pectoralis major—pulls the shoulder down and forward
- Latissimus dorsi—extends upper arm; adducts upper arm posteriorly
- Serratus anterior—pulls the shoulder forward; abducts and rotates it upward
- Subscapularis—rotates the upper arm in toward center of torso
- Supraspinatus—assists in abducting arm
- Teres major—assists in extension, adduction, and medial rotation of arm
- Teres minor—rotates arm outward
- Infraspinatus—rotates arm outward

Dumbbells play a vital role in deltoid development. In fact, only your biceps require more frequent use of dumbbell exercises than do your deltoids. There are more than two dozen highly effective deltoid- and trapezius-developing movements in this chapter. Dive in deep enough and you can skip the tailor's padding.

Barbell Press

Muscles Involved
Overhead pressing movements involve all three deltoid muscles (anterior, lateral, and posterior) along with the rotator cuff muscles (supraspinatus, infraspinatus, teres minor, and subscapularis). Secondary work is performed by latissimus dorsi, pectoralis major, trapezius, triceps, and biceps. The erector spinae muscles are intensely involved as stabilizers.

Position
Wear your lifting belt. Use a power rack or other weight support rack from which to take the bar. Adjust the rack so that the bar is

just below the top of your shoulders. Load the plates onto the bar, being certain to secure each end with collars.

With a shoulder-width stance, place a moderately heavy barbell across the top of your chest with hands and wrists under the

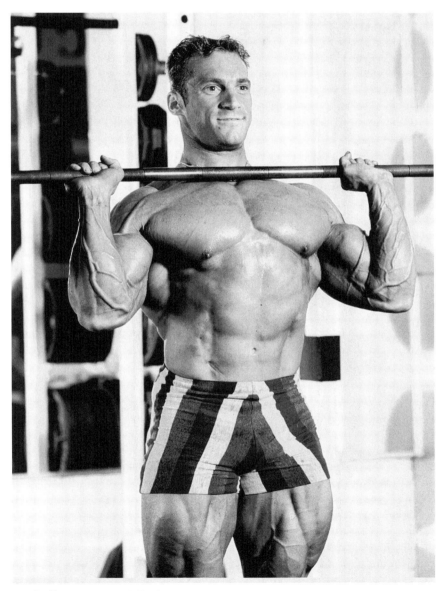

Barbell Press Remi Zuri

bar in a wider-than-your-shoulders grip. Step back with the bar across the top of your chest and shoulders. Take a slightly-less-than-shoulder-width stance to perform the exercise. Maintain an erect posture during the entire movement.

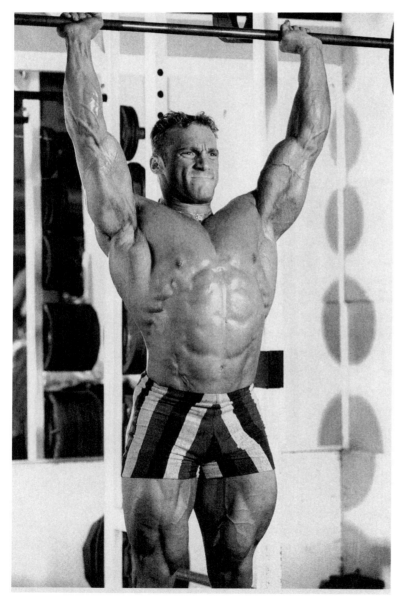

Barbell Press Remi Zuri

Movement Performance
Without allowing your torso to bend backward, slowly push the bar directly upward, close to your face until it is at straight arm's length directly overhead. Lower the bar slowly back to the starting point without any type of bouncing and repeat for the desired number of reps.

Tips
Many benches have been specially designed for performing this movement from a seated Barbell Press. A Smith Machine apparatus may also be used.

Dumbbell Press

Muscles Involved
Overhead pressing movements involve all three deltoid muscles (anterior, lateral, and posterior) along with the rotator cuff muscles (supraspinatus, infraspinatus, teres minor, and subscapularis).
Secondary work is performed

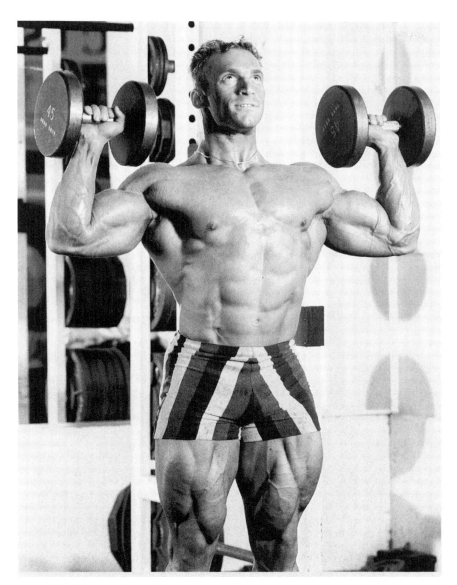

Dumbbell Press Remi Zuri

by latissimus dorsi, pectoralis major, trapezius, triceps, and biceps. The erector spinae muscles are intensely involved as stabilizers. Due to the independent movement of the arms as compared to Barbell Presses, additional work is performed by all the stabilizing muscles.

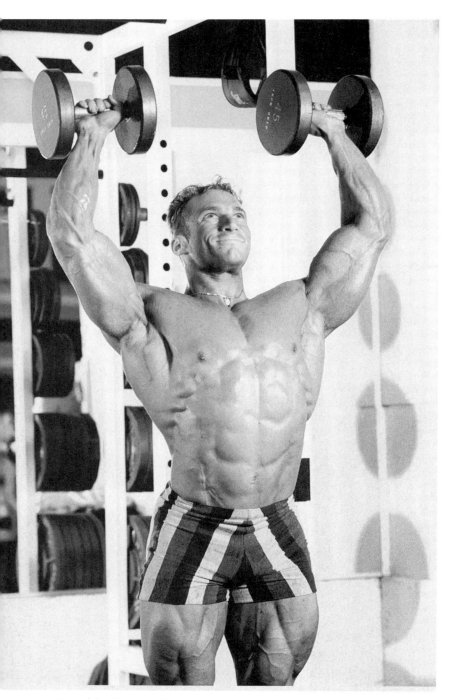

Dumbbell Press Remi Zuri

Position

Wear your lifting belt. With a shoulder-width stance, grab a set of moderately heavy dumbbells from their racks and take a step back. With a controlled swing, bring the dumbbells to a position where your palms are facing away from your torso with the inside plates at the outer edge of your lateral deltoid.

Movement Performance

Without allowing your torso to bend backward, slowly press the dumbbells directly overhead. Do not firmly lock your elbows at the top of the movement. From this almost straight-arm position, reverse the movement and slowly lower the dumbbells back to the bottom point. Repeat for the desired number of reps.

Machine Press

Muscles Involved

Overhead pressing movements involve all three deltoid muscles (anterior, lateral, and posterior) along with the rotator cuff muscles (supraspinatus, infraspinatus, teres minor, and subscapularis). Secondary work is performed by latissimus dorsi, pectoralis major, trapezius, triceps, and biceps. There is near total deltoid isolation designed into the latest generation of Machine Press equipment. The ability to cheat during the exercise is removed.

Position
Set the resistance on the machine to an appropriate amount. Adjust the height of the seat so that your hands, when in the bottom pressing position, are just above the machine's handles.

Movement Performance
Sit in the machine and lock yourself in position. Take a just-beyond-shoulder-width grip on the handles. Grasping the handles and sitting erect, the resistance should be engaged and held in the starting position. Slowly straighten your arms, raising them to a point straight over your head. Then reverse the motion to the initial starting point and repeat for the desired rep count.

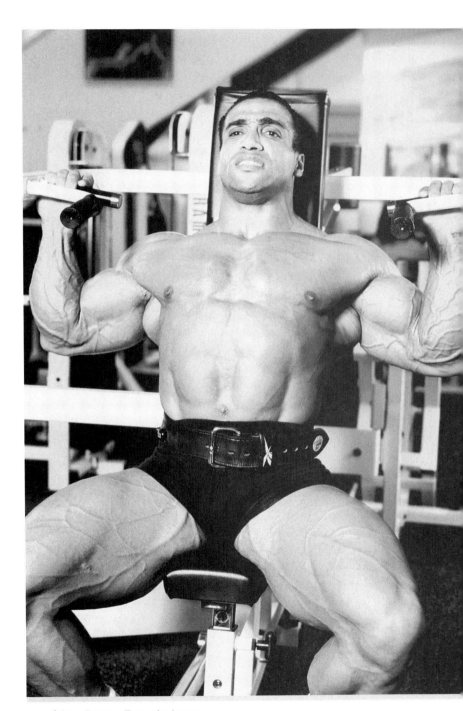

Machine Press Dennis James

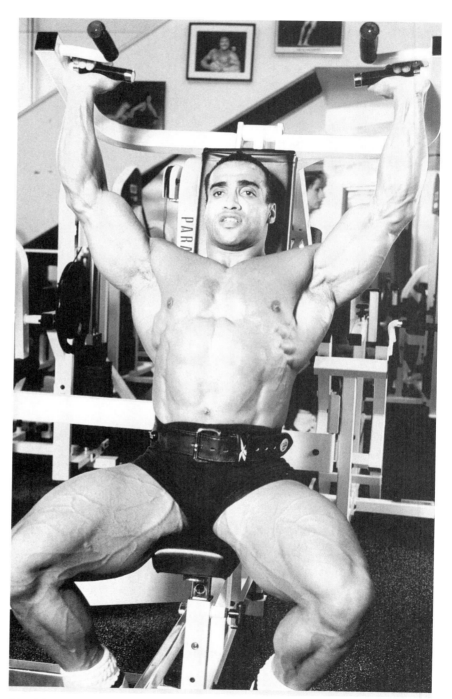

Machine Press Dennis James

Seated Smith Machine Press Behind the Neck

Muscles Involved

Overhead pressing movements involve all three deltoid muscles (anterior, lateral, and posterior) along with the rotator cuff muscles (supraspinatus, infraspinatus, teres minor, and subscapularis). Secondary work is performed by latissimus dorsi, pectoralis major, trapezius, triceps, and biceps. There is near total deltoid isolation designed into the latest generation of Smith Machines.

Position

Set the bench at an angle just short of 90 degrees. Position it so that the seat is directly underneath the bar. Set the bar at a height so that when you are seated, it is just below your extended arms' length. Load the plates onto the bar. Sit down on the seat and place your hands slightly wider than shoulder width with your palms facing away from you. Make certain that your back is stable and slightly arched.

Movement Performance

With a firm grip on the bar, press upward to release the

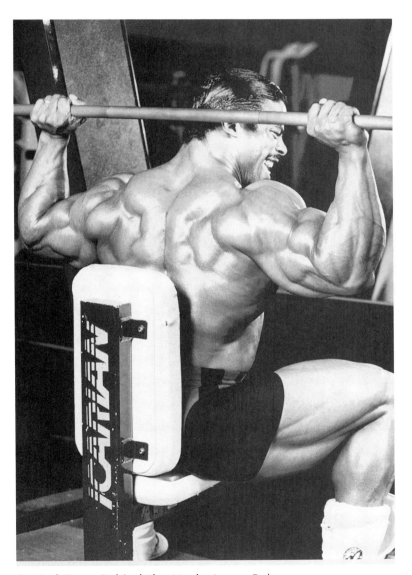

Seated Press Behind the Neck Aaron Baker

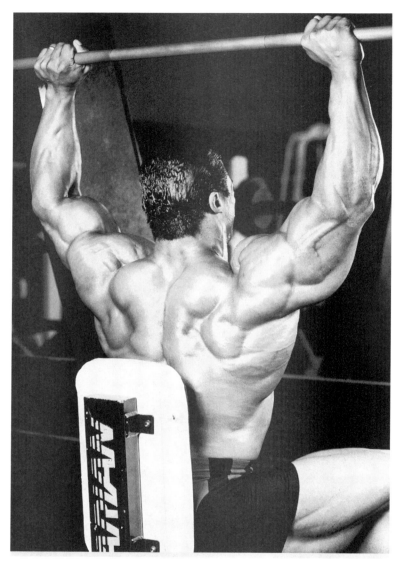

Seated Press Behind the Neck Aaron Baker

spotting hooks on the machine. As your arms fully straighten, rotate the bar backward just enough to be able to clear the safety catches as you lower the bar during the exercise. This is done by pulling your knuckles toward the base of your neck.

With the bar clear of the safety catches, begin to lower it to a position just below the bottom of your ear. You should move your elbows in a path directly underneath the bar. At the bottom point of the exercise your forearms should be close to or actually touching the biceps. From this position reverse your movement and press the bar back up to arms' length.

Seated Dumbbell Press

Muscles Involved
This versatile shoulder movement stresses all three deltoid muscles (anterior, lateral, and posterior) along with the rotator cuff muscles (supraspinatus, infraspinatus, teres minor, and subscapularis). Secondary work is performed by latissimus dorsi, pectoralis major, trapezius, triceps, and biceps. Due to the independent movement of the arms as compared to Barbell Presses, additional work is performed by all the stabilizing muscles.

Position

Wear your belt and grasp two moderately heavy dumbbells. Sit down on a sturdy bench with a supportive back for balance during the movement. Rock the dumbbells from your knees to your shoulders. The palms are to be facing away from your torso. The

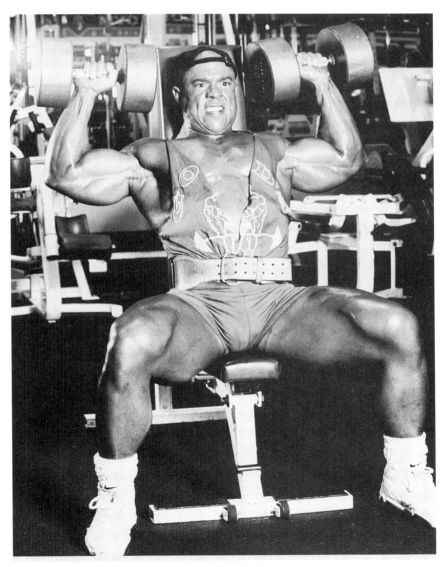

Seated Dumbbell Press Skip LaCour

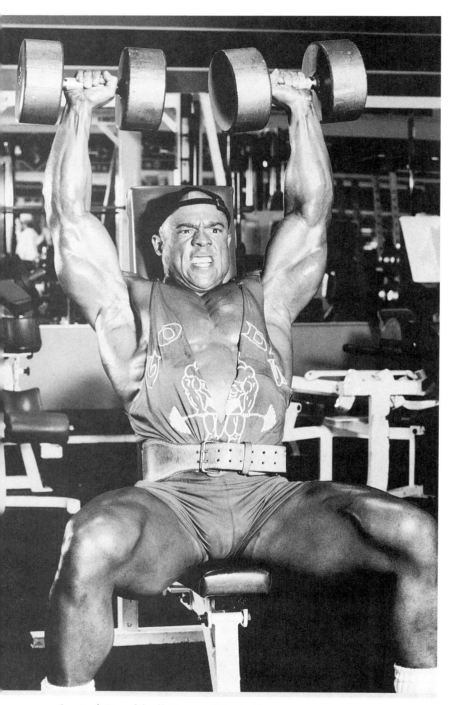

Seated Dumbbell Press Skip LaCour

inside plates should rest lightly on the outer edge of your lateral deltoid. Firmly arch your back and place your feet firmly on the floor.

Movement Performance
With the elbows directly underneath the dumbbells, press them to an overhead position. At the top of the pressing movement the dumbbells should be one to two inches apart above your head. Following the same path of travel lower the dumbbells back to the starting point. Repeat the movement for the correct number of reps.

Tips
The use of dumbbells allows for variety and creativity when planning your workouts. For a change from conventional dumbbell presses, you can press with your palms facing each other instead of away from your body.

Reverse Dumbbell Press

Muscles Involved
This shoulder movement stresses all three deltoid muscles (anterior, lateral, and pos-

terior) along with the rotator cuff muscles (supraspinatus, infraspinatus, teres minor, and subscapularis). In particular the posterior deltoids are heavily involved during the performance of this exercise. Secondary work is performed by latissimus dorsi, pectoralis major, trapezius, triceps, and biceps. Due to the independent movement of the arms as compared to Barbell Presses, additional work is performed by all the stabilizing muscles.

Position
This exercise closely resembles conventional presses. However, you cannot use similar weights. Reverse Presses eliminate much of the shoulder's power, so therefore you need to train with lighter dumbbells.

Wear your belt. Grasp two dumbbells and sit down on a sturdy bench with a supportive back for balance during the movement. Bring the dumbbells to your shoulders and press to an overhead position. Rotate your hands so that the palms face backward toward your body as in curls, for example. The correct starting position is arms overhead with palms facing toward you.

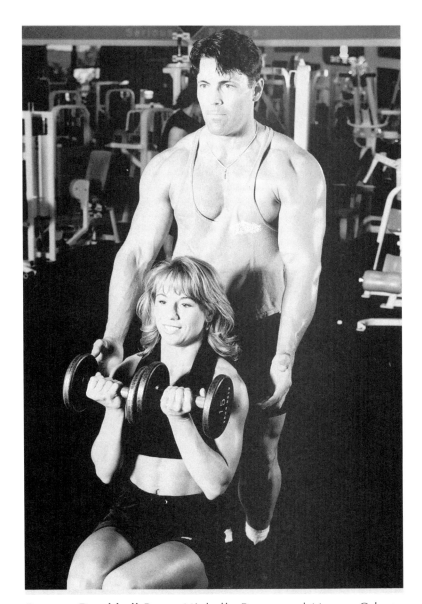

Reverse Dumbbell Press Michelle Brown and Marcus Odum

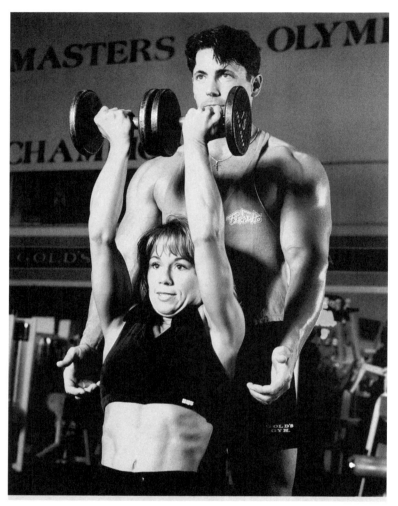

Reverse Dumbbell Press Michelle Brown and Marcus Odum

Movement Performance
With a deliberately slow motion, lower the dumbbells while keeping them no more than two inches apart from each other. Keep your elbows underneath the weights and allow them to move backward from the sides of your torso.

The bottom position is with the dumbbells resting in front of your upper chest. Keep the dumbbells close together and press back to arms' length overhead. Drive in an upward motion with your elbows. Repeat for the desired number of reps.

The most difficult portion of the movement is the lowering of the dumbbells with resistance provided by your posterior deltoids.

Tip
A barbell can be used as an alternative to dumbbells. Some bodybuilders find it easier to use a barbell when first attempting this movement. It is a matter of trial and error.

Reverse-Grip Barbell Front Raise

Muscles Involved
Reverse-Grip Barbell Front Raises effectively isolate the anterior deltoids. Major involvement of the posterior and lateral deltoids

also occurs. The secondary muscle groups involved are the same as for the overhead pressing exercises described previously in this chapter.

Position

Wear your lifting belt. Ideally this exercise is performed with a four-foot-long, pre-set barbell as shown in the illustration. The reversing of the grip to a palms up position decreases the functional leverage and therefore heavy weights are not required. The starting position is a shoulder-width stance, barbell held palms up with your hands at the outside edge of your upper thighs, and looking straight ahead.

Movement Performance

Stand tall with a slight arch in your lower back. Without bending your arms, raise the barbell to a point an inch or two above your shoulders. From the uppermost elevation, slowly reverse the motion back to the starting point. Pay particular attention to the

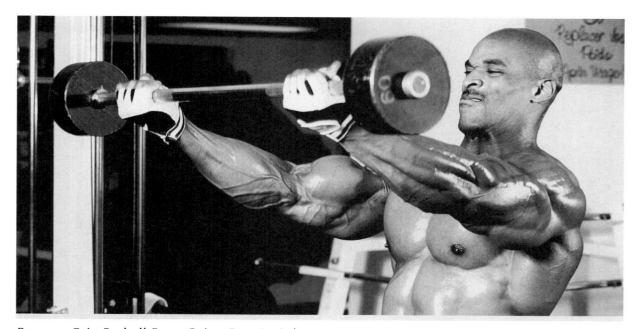

Reverse-Grip Barbell Front Raise Ronnie Coleman

lowering of the weight because the downward aspect is vital to achieving maximum results from this effective movement. Repeat for the desired number of reps.

Machine Rear Lateral

Muscles Involved
This movement allows you to isolate stress on your posterior deltoids with minimal involvement of the anterior and lateral deltoids. The trapezius, latissimus dorsi, rhomboideus major, teres major and minor, and triceps muscles all perform secondary work.

Position
Adjust the seat to a height that puts your shoulders in line with the handles on the machine. Sit facing the pad. Place your torso

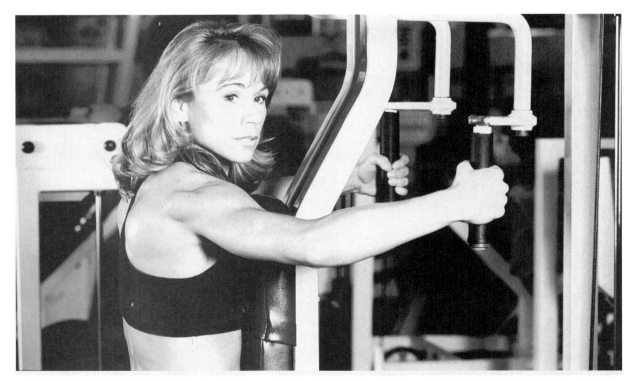

Machine Rear Lateral Michelle Brown

firmly against the pad and place your hands on the gripping area. Raise your elbows so that they are in line with your shoulders and hands. Maintain a partial bend at the elbow.

Movement Performance

Keeping your elbows bent, squeeze your shoulder blades together as firmly as possible. From this position draw your hands backward and behind you. Keep your shoulder blades pinched together.

At the point of maximum contraction, reverse the movement and slowly allow the resistance to draw your hands back to their original position. Repeat for the desired number of reps.

Pay particular attention to the lowering of the weight. The downward movement is vital to achieving maximum results from this effective exercise.

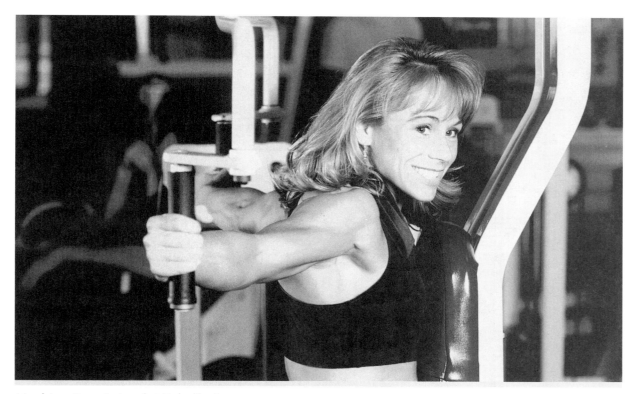

Machine Rear Lateral Michelle Brown

Seated Dumbbell Rear Raise

Muscles Involved
This movement allows you to isolate stress on your posterior
deltoids with minimal involvement of the anterior and lateral
deltoids. The trapezius,
latissimus dorsi, rhomboideus
major, teres major and minor,
and triceps muscles all perform secondary work.

Position
Grasp two light dumbbells and
sit at the end of a flat bench,
facing away from the length of
the bench. Place your feet
close to each other about two
feet out from the end of the
bench.

Bend over at the waist
and rest your torso along your
thighs, with your arms
pointed directly down toward
the floor. Your palms are to
face each other. Bend your
elbows slightly and maintain
this position throughout the
movement.

Movement Performance
Without moving your torso,
slowly raise the dumbbells in
semicircular arcs directly out
at your sides until they are at
shoulder level. Lower the
dumbbells slowly back to the

Seated Dumbbell Rear Raise Aaron Baker

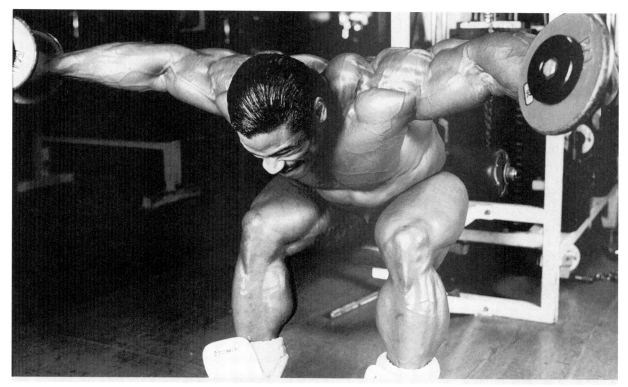

Seated Dumbbell Rear Raise Aaron Baker

starting point and repeat for the desired rep count. Do not allow
your torso to move from its starting position.

Tip
For a unique stress on your posterior deltoids, you can raise the
dumbbells slightly forward as you raise them out to the sides.

Cable Rear Raise

Muscles Involved
This movement allows you to isolate stress on your posterior deltoids with minimal involvement of the anterior and lateral deltoids. The trapezius, latissimus dorsi, rhomboideus major, teres

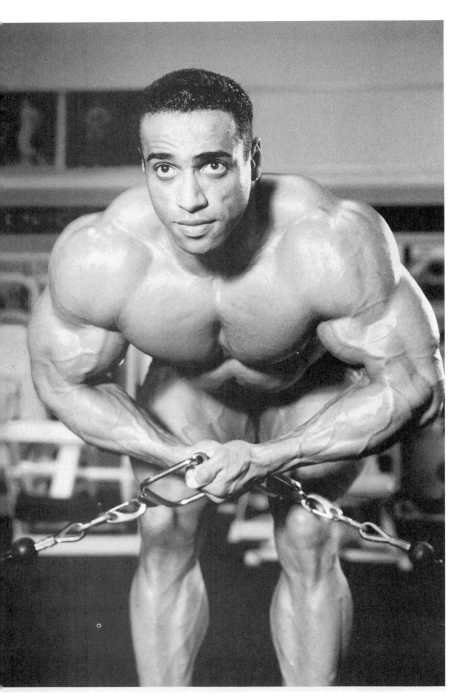

Cable Rear Raise Aaron Baker

major and minor, and triceps muscles all perform secondary work.

Position
Place the handles on the floor between the poles of the equipment. Stand between the handles. Bend forward at the waist with your back arched. Bend your knees, reach down to grab the left handle with your right hand and the right handle with your left hand.

Straighten your knees so that the handles draw the cables tight against the weight stack. Your hands should be crossed approximately in front of your knees. Your palms are to face each other. Bend your elbows slightly and maintain this position throughout the movement.

Movement Performance
Without moving your torso, slowly raise the handles in semicircular arcs directly out at your sides until they are at shoulder level. Squeeze your shoulder blades together at the point of maximum con-traction. Slowly lower the handles back to the starting point and repeat for the

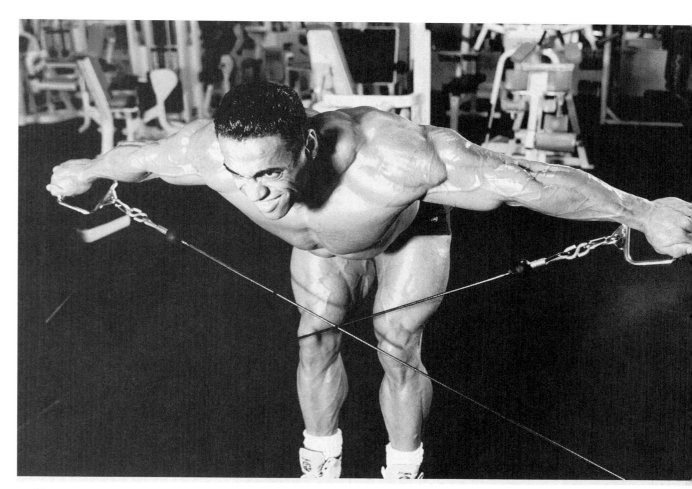

Cable Rear Raise Aaron Baker

desired rep count. Do not allow your torso to move from its starting position.

One-Arm Machine Side Lateral

Muscles Involved
In particular the lateral deltoids are effectively isolated during the
performance of this exercise. As with all the variations of laterals,

this versatile shoulder movement stresses all three deltoid muscles (anterior, lateral, and posterior) along with the rotator cuff muscles (supraspinatus, infraspinatus, teres minor, and subscapularis). Secondary work is performed by latissimus dorsi, pectoralis major, trapezius, triceps, and biceps.

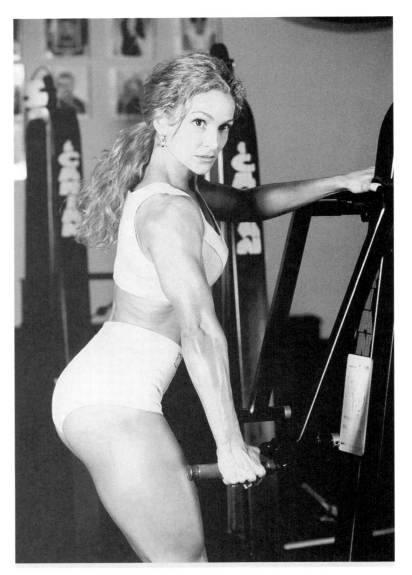

One-Arm Machine Side Lateral Mia Finnegan

Position

Stand in front of the machine with the right handle at the outside edge of your right thigh. Place your left hand on the area provided and arch your back. Reach down and grab the right handle with your right hand. Straighten your upper body so that the resistance is felt against the handle.

Movement Performance

Without moving your torso, slowly raise the handle in a semicircular arc directly out to your side until it is at shoulder level. Keep your arm relatively straight throughout the movement.

From the highest point, reverse the motion in a path back to the starting point. Make sure to lower the weight slowly and under complete control. Repeat for the desired number of repetitions and then switch to your left side and perform for a complete set.

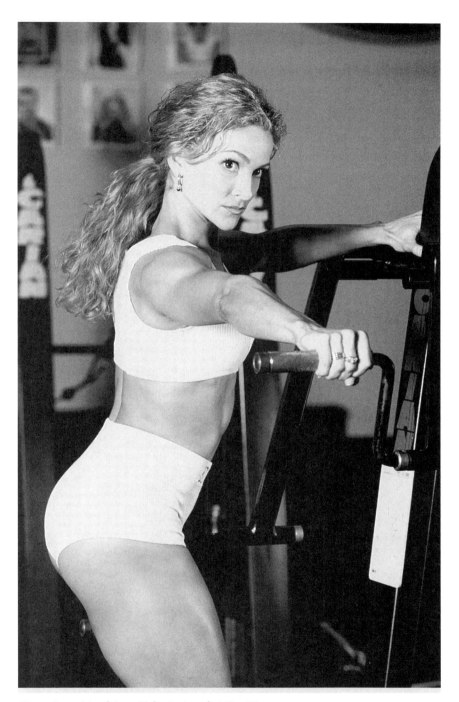

One-Arm Machine Side Lateral Mia Finnegan

Cable Side Lateral

Muscles Involved
In particular the lateral deltoids are effectively isolated during the performance of this exercise. As with all the variations of shoulder raises or laterals, this versatile shoulder movement

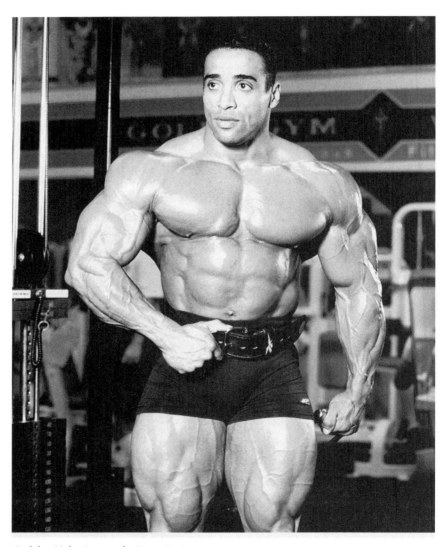

Cable Side Lateral Dennis James

stresses all three deltoid muscles (anterior, lateral, and posterior) along with the rotator cuff muscles (supraspinatus, infraspinatus, teres minor, and subscapularis). Secondary work is performed by latissimus dorsi, pectoralis major, trapezius, triceps, and biceps.

Position
Attach the handle to the low pulley and place on the floor. Stand with your right shoulder about 6–8 inches from the weight stack, with the cable and handles behind your heels. Squat down and with your left hand grab the handle. Stand erect with the cable behind you and the handle at the outside edge of your left thigh. Brace yourself with your right hand; keep your knees slightly bent and your back arched.

Movement Performance
Without moving your torso, slowly raise the handle in a semicircular arc directly out to your side until it is at shoulder level. Keep your arm relatively straight throughout the movement.

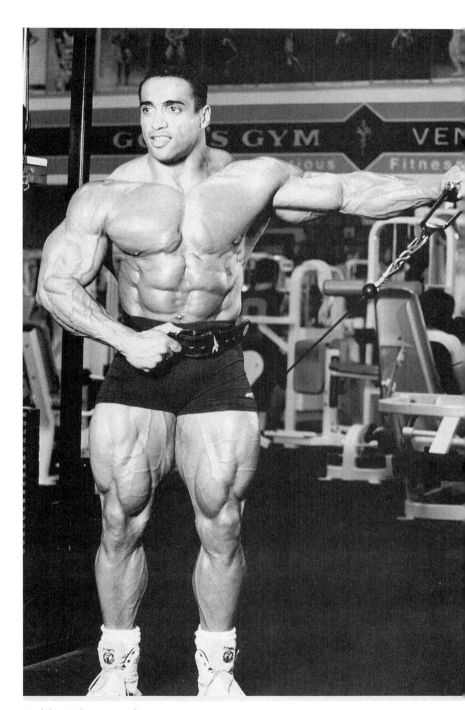

Cable Side Lateral Dennis James

From the highest point, reverse the motion in a path back to the starting point. Make sure to lower the weight slowly and under complete control. Repeat for the desired number of repetitions and then switch to your right side and perform for a complete set.

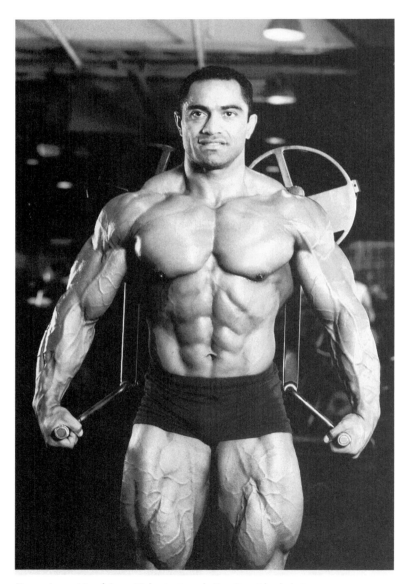

Two-Arm Machine Side Lateral Tevita Aholelei

Two-Arm Machine Side Lateral

Muscles Involved
In particular the lateral deltoids are effectively isolated during the performance of this exercise. As with all the variations of laterals, this versatile shoulder movement stresses all three deltoid muscles (anterior, lateral, and posterior) along with the rotator cuff muscles (supraspinatus, infraspinatus, teres minor, and subscapularis). Secondary work is performed by latissimus dorsi, pectoralis major, trapezius, triceps, and biceps.

Position
Stand between the handles, facing away from the weight stack. The handles should be at the outside of your thighs. With your back arched, squat down to grab the handles with your hands. Stand up straight so that the resistance

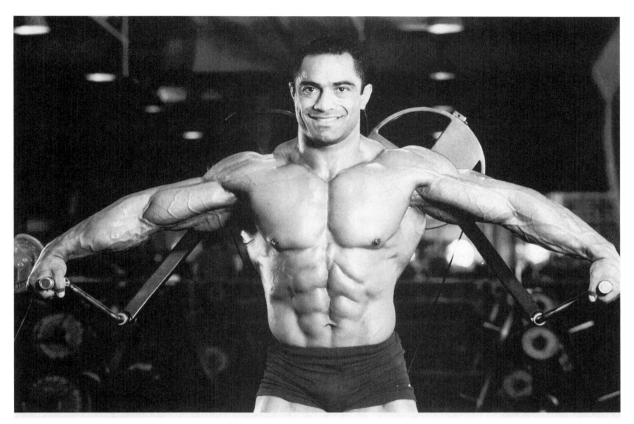

Two-Arm Machine Side Lateral Tevita Aholelei

is felt against the handles. Your shoulder joints should be aligned with the pivot points of each side of the machine. These are the centers of rotation around which the movement occurs on the equipment.

Movement Performance
Moving only your arms, and with your elbows straight, raise the handles in a semicircular arc directly out to your sides until they are at shoulder level. Keep your arms relatively straight throughout the movement.

From the highest point, reverse the motion in a path back to the starting point. Make sure to lower the weight slowly and under complete control. Repeat for the desired number of repetitions.

Tip
An alternative to the above type of Two-Arm Machine Lateral is performed on equipment with wide pads (instead of handles) that allows the resistance to be moved with your elbows as opposed to your hands.

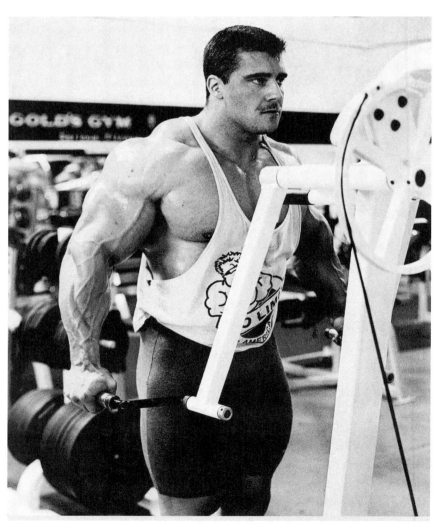

Two-Arm Machine Side Lateral Jean-Pierre Fux

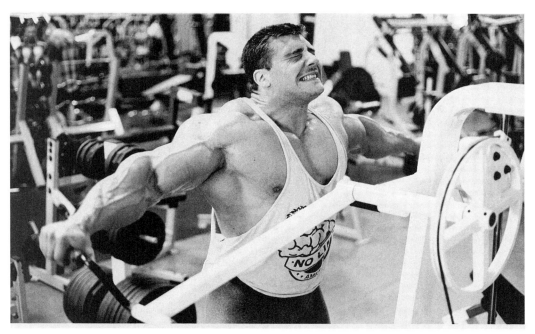

Two-Arm Machine Side Lateral Jean-Pierre Fux

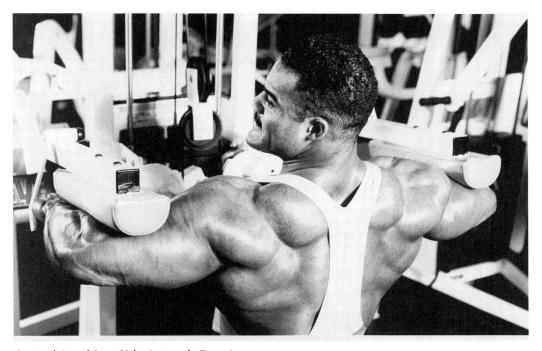

Seated Machine Side Lateral Don Long

Side Dumbbell Raise

Muscles Involved
This movement is often incorrectly performed. Correctly executed, Side Dumbbell Raises stress the lateral heads of the deltoids in near total isolation. As with all the variations of laterals, this versatile shoulder movement stresses all three deltoid muscles (anterior, lateral, and posterior) along with the rotator cuff muscles (supraspinatus, infraspinatus, teres minor, and subscapularis). Secondary work is performed by latissimus dorsi, pectoralis major, trapezius, triceps, and biceps.

Position
Wear your lifting belt. Grasp two dumbbells, place your feet about shoulder width apart, and stand erect. Bend slightly forward at the waist and press the dumbbells together, palms facing each other, in front of your hips. Keep your arms straight throughout the movement.

Movement Performance
Using deltoid strength and keeping your palms toward the floor throughout the movement, raise the dumbbells in semicircular arcs out to the sides and slightly forward until they are just above the level of your shoulders. Once you have raised the dumbbells to shoulder level, lower them slowly back along the same arc to the starting point and repeat the movement for the desired number of reps.

Tip
To obtain even more deltoid isolation you can perform this movement while seated at the end of a sturdy bench (known as Seated Side Dumbbell Raise). From the seated position, you start the movement with the dumbbells resting just below your hips, arms directly at your sides. Raise the dumbbells to shoulder level and then lower slowly to the starting position.

Dumbbell Raise—45-Degree Front

Muscles Involved

This dumbbell raise, due to the 45-degree angle of the dumbbells relative to the front of your torso, stresses both the anterior and lateral deltoids. As with all the variations of laterals, this versatile shoulder movement stresses all three deltoid muscles (anterior, lateral, and posterior) along with the rotator cuff muscles (supraspinatus, infraspinatus, teres minor, and subscapularis). Secondary work is performed by latissimus dorsi, pectoralis major, trapezius, triceps, and biceps.

Position

Wear your lifting belt. Grasp two dumbbells, place your feet about shoulder width apart, and stand erect. Bend slightly forward at the waist and press the dumbbells together, palms facing each other, in front of your hips. Keep your arms straight throughout the movement.

Movement Performance

Instead of raising your arms in front of you, move them approximately halfway between directly to your side and directly to the front. At shoulder level, your arms are in a V shape.

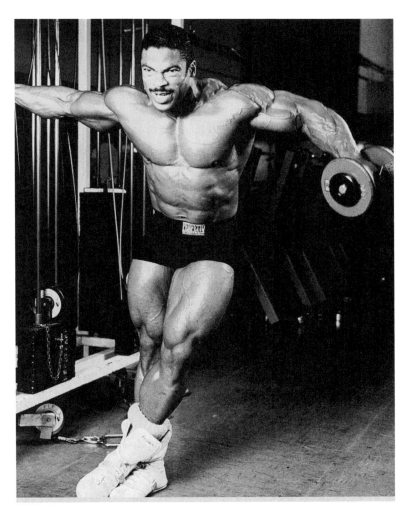

One-Arm Dumbbell Side Raise Aaron Baker

Combination Front/Side Dumbbell Raise

Muscles Involved
A dual level of stress is placed on the anterior and medial deltoid heads.

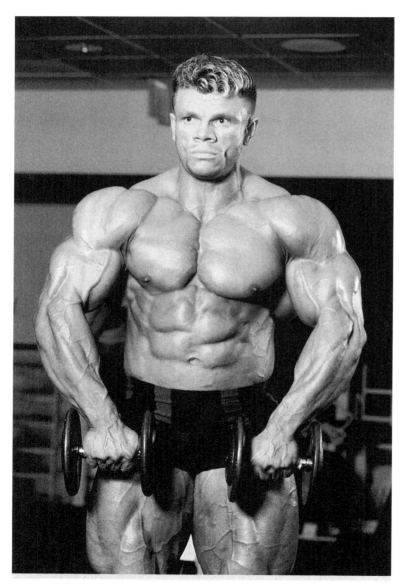

Front Dumbbell Raise Roland Cziurlok

Position
Wear your lifting belt. Grasp two dumbbells, place your feet about shoulder width apart, and stand erect. Bend slightly forward at the waist and press the dumbbells together, palms facing each other, in front of your hips. Keep your arms straight throughout the movement.

Movement Performance
First perform a conventional dumbbell side raise (rep #1) and upon reaching the starting position, immediately perform a conventional dumbbell front raise (rep #2). Alternate between raises to the side and raises to the front. Repeat in this fashion until desired number of reps are finished.

Front Dumbbell Raise

Muscles Involved
When correctly executed, Dumbbell Raises to the Front

stress the anterior heads of the deltoids in near total isolation. As
with all the variations of laterals, this versatile shoulder movement stresses all three deltoid
muscles (anterior, lateral, and
posterior) along with the rotator cuff muscles (supraspinatus, infraspinatus, teres
minor, and subscapularis).
Secondary work is performed
by latissimus dorsi, pectoralis
major, trapezius, triceps, and
biceps.

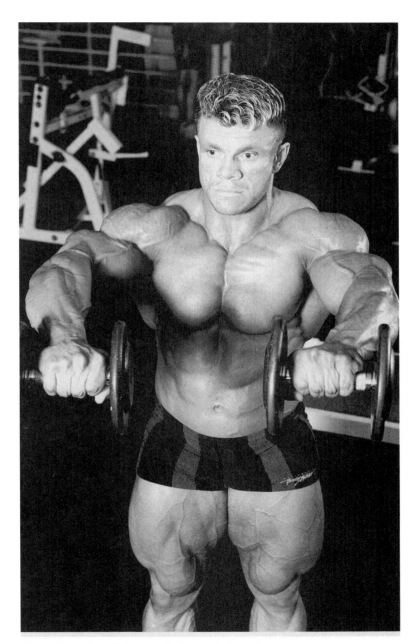

Position
Grasp a pair of dumbbells and
stand erect with your palms
facing the fronts of your
thighs. The two dumbbells
should be approximately 4–6
inches apart. Set your feet
about shoulder width apart
and look straight ahead. Keep
your arms straight throughout the movement.

Movement Performance
Moving just your arms, slowly
raise the dumbbells in a semicircular arc from your thighs
to the height of your shoulders. From the position at
shoulder level, slowly lower
the dumbbells back to the
starting position and repeat
for the desired number of
reps.

Front Dumbbell Raise Roland Cziurlok

One-Arm Cable Front Raise

Muscles Involved

This exercise isolates the anterior deltoids. As with other types of cable shoulder movements, this movement stresses all three deltoid muscles (anterior, lateral, and posterior) along with the rotator cuff muscles (supraspinatus, infraspinatus, teres minor, and subscapularis).

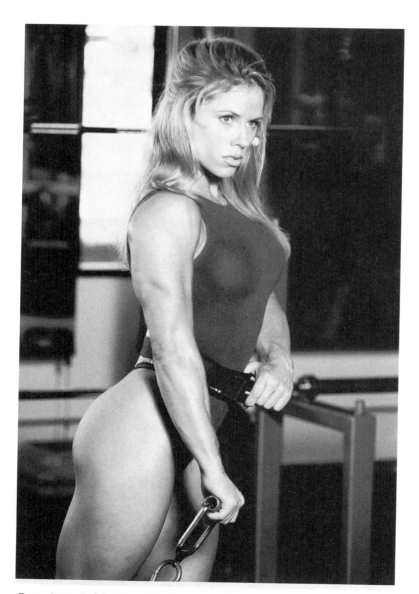

Position

Wear your lifting belt. Attach a handle to a low cable pulley. Stand with your right foot next to the handle on the cable. Face away from the weight stack. Bend down and grab the handle with your right hand. The handle should be next to your right thigh in the starting position. Stand erect with your back arched and your left hand braced for support. You may perform this exercise with your feet set apart as shown in the illustration or with your heels together.

Movement Performance

Moving just your arms, slowly raise the handle in a semicircular arc from your thigh to the height of your shoulders. Keep your arm straight during

One-Arm Cable Front Raise Monica Brant

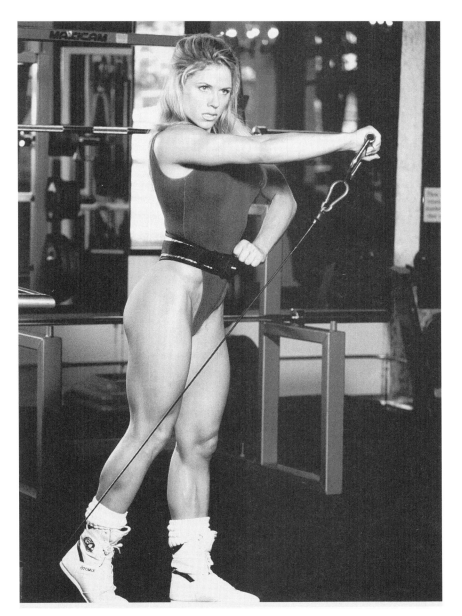

One-Arm Cable Front Raise Monica Brant

the movement. From the position at shoulder level, slowly lower
the handle back to the starting position and repeat for the desired
number of reps. When you have completed with your right side,
switch position for the left side and continue for a complete set.

Incline Dumbbell Raise

Muscles Involved
As with all the variations of laterals, this versatile shoulder move-ment stresses all three deltoid muscles (anterior, lateral, and posterior) along with the rotator cuff muscles (supraspinatus, infraspinatus, teres minor, and subscapularis). Secondary work is performed by latissimus dorsi, pectoralis major, trapezius, triceps, and biceps.

Position
Grasp a light dumbbell in your left hand and lie on your right side on a 30-to-45-degree incline bench. Bend your arm slightly throughout the movement. Allow the weight of the dumbbell to pull your left hand to the level of the bench, if not 1–2 inches below.

Movement Performance
Slowly raise the dumbbell directly out to the side and upward in a semicircular arc until it is directly above your left shoulder joint. Lower the weight back to the starting point and repeat the move-ment. Switch sides on the bench and repeat for your right shoul-der. Be sure to complete an equal number of reps for each arm.

Barbell Upright Row

Muscles Involved
All variations of the Upright Row significantly impact the trape-zius, posterior, anterior, and lateral deltoids, biceps, brachialis, forearm flexors, supraspinatus, infraspinatus, teres minor, and subscapularis muscles. Secondary work is performed by latissimus dorsi, pectoralis major, and triceps.

Position
Wear your belt. Take a narrow overhand grip in the middle of a barbell about 6 inches between index fingers. Stand erect with your arms straight down at your sides and your fists resting on your upper thighs.

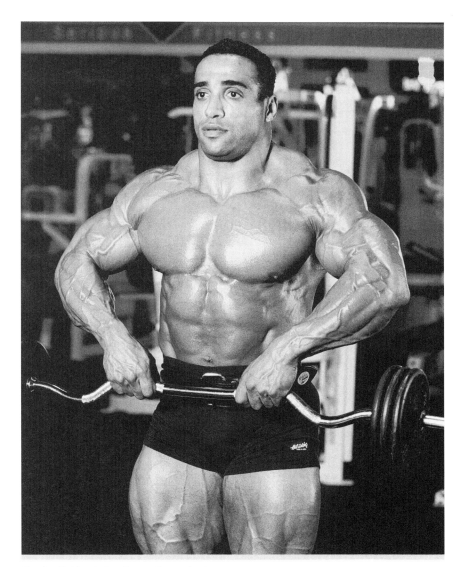

Barbell Upright Row Dennis James

Movement Performance
Being sure to keep your elbows well above the level of your grip
on the bar at all times, slowly pull the barbell directly upward
close to your body until your palms are shoulder level.

In the top position, roll your shoulders backward and
squeeze your shoulder blades together. Lower the weight slowly

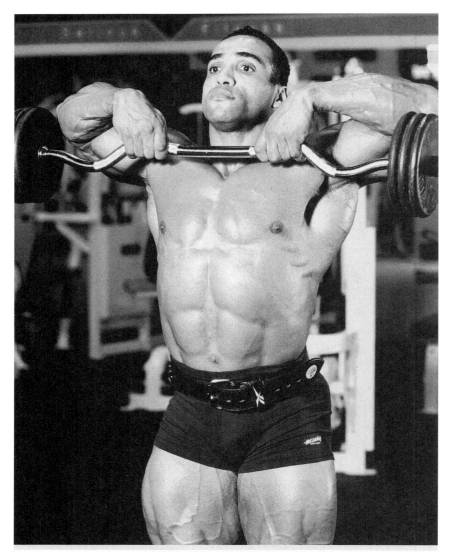

Barbell Upright Row Dennis James

back to the starting point and repeat for the desired number of reps.

Tip
Moving your grip outward to various degrees allows the same muscles to be stressed in different ways.

SHOULDER AND TRAPEZIUS TRAINING

Dumbbell Upright Row

Muscles Involved
Dumbbells give you somewhat more freedom of movement than a barbell when you're performing Upright Rows. All variations of the Upright Row significantly impact the trapezius, deltoids (posterior, anterior, and lateral), biceps, brachialis, forearm flexors, supraspinatus, infraspinatus, teres minor, and subscapularis muscles. Secondary work is performed by latissimus dorsi, pectoralis major, and triceps.

Position
Wear your belt. Grasp two moderately heavy dumbbells and stand erect with your arms hanging straight down, your palms facing the front of your body, and the dumbbells resting across your upper thighs.

Movement Performance
Being sure to keep your elbows well above the level of your hands, slowly pull the dumbbells directly upward along the front of your body until they are just below your lower pectorals.

Lower the dumbbells slowly and deliberately back to the starting position and continue the movement until you complete the desired number of reps.

Tip
This type of rowing motion also can be performed with a low cable pulley machine. A narrow straight pulley handle bar about 12 inches in length works well.

Barbell Shrug

Muscles Involved
Barbell Shrugs are a direct movement for stressing the trapezius and other upper back muscles. Secondary stress is on the gripping muscles of your forearms.

Position
Wear your lifting belt. Assume a standing position in front of a power rack with the pins set so that the level of the bar is at the tip of your fingers. Set your feet firmly on the floor slightly less than shoulder width apart.

Grasp the bar at a width so that your hands are touching the outside edge of your legs. Use a thumbs-around-the-back grip with your palms facing away. Use straps if your grip is insufficient. Raise your head upward, while arching your back.

Movement Performance
Stand up with your legs straight, your back tightly arched, and your head up. Once you are powerfully upright, allow your shoulders to relax. Then pull them upward and slightly to the back, or in other words, just shrug your shoulders up high.

Do not bend forward or lean backward. Keep your lower back arched. Squeeze at the top for peak contraction. Reverse the movement and repeat for the desired repetition count.

Tip
Widening or narrowing your grip creates different angles to challenge the area.

Dumbbell Shrug

Muscles Involved
The Dumbbell Shrug is another direct movement for stressing the trapezius and other upper back muscles. Secondary stress is on the gripping muscles of the forearms.

You will have more mobility in the shoulders when using a pair of dumbbells, so in some ways Dumbbell Shrugs are superior to Barbell Shrugs.

Position
Wear your lifting belt. Grasp two heavy dumbbells, assume the basic pulling position and lift the weights up to the front of your

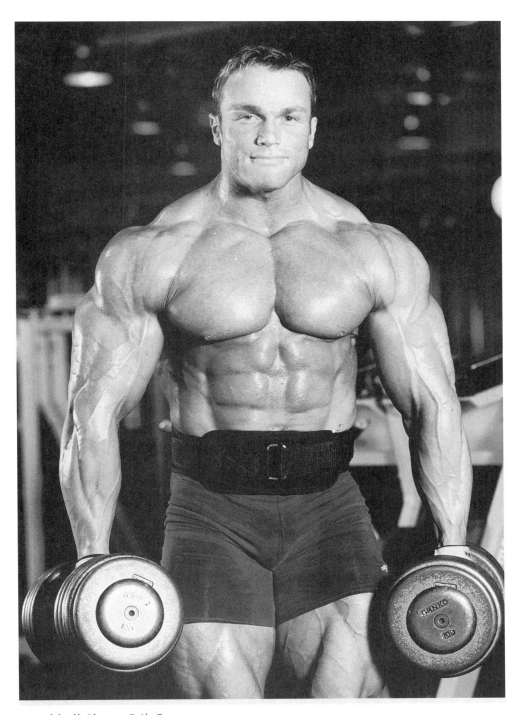

Dumbbell Shrug Erik Fromm

thighs. Hold your arms straight and your torso securely erect. Allow your shoulders to relax and sag downward as far as comfortable.

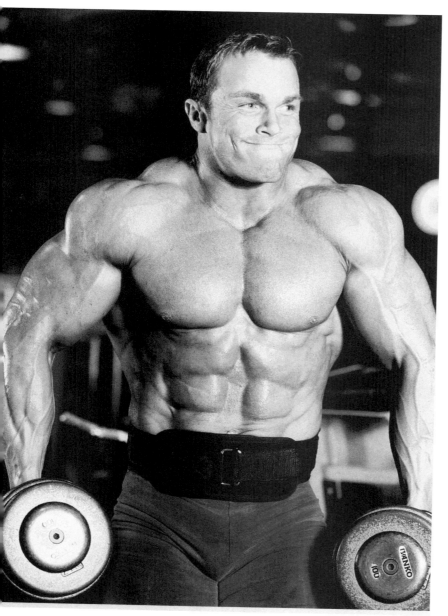

Dumbbell Shrug Erik Fromm

Movement Performance
Slowly shrug your shoulders upward and backward as far as possible. Hold this peak-contracted top position for a moment, then lower the dumbbells back to the starting point. Repeat for the desired number of reps.

Tip
Rotating your shoulders around in a semicircular shrug adds variation to this effective movement.

Seated Hammer Shrug (Machine Shrug)

Muscles Involved
As with all shrug-type movements, shrugs performed on specially designed benches or machines place tremendous primary stress on the trapezius and other upper back muscles. Secondary stress is felt by the forearm flexor muscles.

Position
Elevate the seat height so that when your arms are resting at

your sides, your hands are slightly above the level of the gripping handles.

Keep your back arched firmly and head elevated throughout the entire movement. Wear a lifting belt. Lean forward and grasp the handles firmly, then sit up straight.

Movement Performance
Slowly allow your shoulders to be pulled downward to a maximum comfortable stretch. At the bottom point of the stretch begin to slowly shrug upward and backward as high as possible and hold for a peak contraction. Repeat for the desired number of repetitions.

Lying Rotator Warm-Up

Muscles Involved
This is a great exercise to adopt as a favorite in your early training years. The muscular imbalance that occurs within the rotator cuff muscles (supraspinatus, infra-

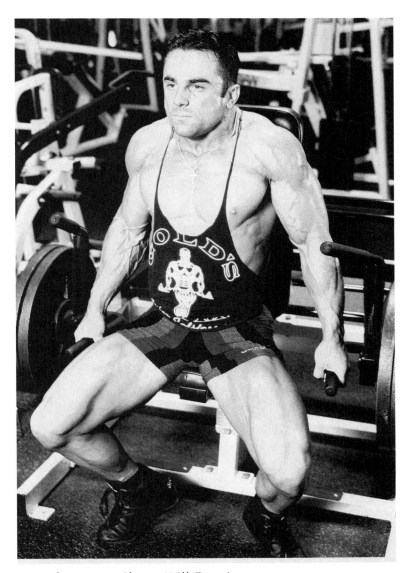

Seated Hammer Shrug Will Duggin

spinatus, teres minor, and subscapularis) is remediated through the performance of this exercise. The weights used in this movement are by necessity light. The ideal degree of isolation that occurs within the rotator cuff muscle group makes this a great choice as one of your regular deltoid exercises.

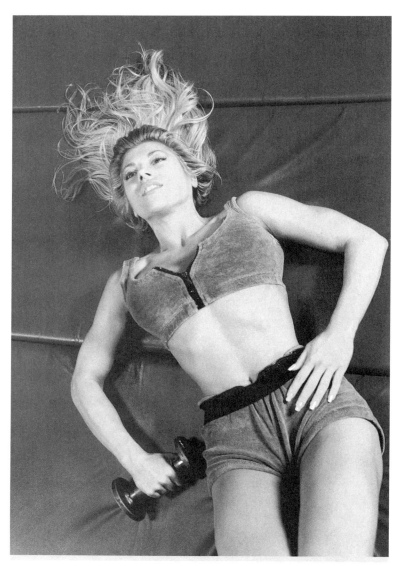

Lying Rotator Warm-Up Jennifer Stimac

Position
Place a light dumbbell (2.5–10 lbs.) on the floor. Lie flat on the floor and place your left arm directly out from your shoulder, forming a straight line. The right arm can be used for balance. Bend your knees slightly with your feet flat on the floor.

Grasp the dumbbell with your left hand and bend your arm down toward your side at a 90-degree angle. The objective in this exercise is to rotate your upper arm upward from the floor toward the ceiling. To start the movement correctly, your upper arm must be in a straight line directly out from the shoulder and your elbow must be bent 90 degrees, palm toward your feet with dumbbell in hand.

Movement Performance
Moving only your hand and forearm, raise the dumbbell till your forearm is in a vertical position, 90 degrees from the starting point. Do not move the dumbbell beyond this point or you risk injury. Be careful to perform this exercise with a slow controlled motion and avoid any fast movements. Repeat for the desired repetition count. Reverse the position so that the dumbbell is on your right side and repeat until both arms are completed.

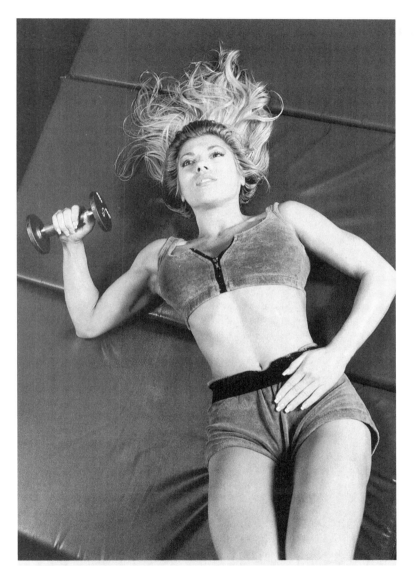

Lying Rotator Warm-Up Jennifer Stimac

Side Bench Rotator Warm-Up

Muscles Involved
This is another invaluable movement to adopt as a shoulder favorite.

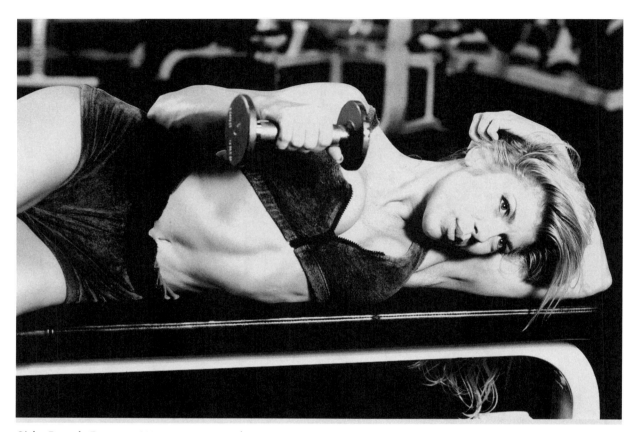

Side Bench Rotator Warm-Up Jennifer Stimac

Position

Place a light dumbbell (2.5–10 pounds) next to a supine (flat) bench. Lie on the bench in the following position: your left arm placed under your head as you lie on your left side, your right leg placed on top of your left leg, and both knees bent. Reach down and grasp the dumbbell with your right hand. Draw your right arm back into a position where your right elbow is bent 90 degrees and your upper arm lies along the side of your torso. This allows the dumbbell and your right palm to face toward your abs.

Movement Performance

Moving only your right hand, lift the dumbbell up toward the ceiling until your forearm is straight up and down. Do not move the dumbbell beyond this point or you risk injury. From this position, slowly allow the dumbbell to return to the starting point next to your abs. Repeat for the desired number of repetitions. Switch sides and repeat for the left arm. Remember to use light weights at all times in all rotator-specific exercises.

Grymko Radical Rack Delt Chin

Muscles Involved
This radical movement involves all three deltoid muscles (anterior, lateral, and posterior) along with the latissimus dorsi, biceps, and trapezius.

Position
Stand facing a power rack with pins at just below the top of your reach with your arms over your head. Grab the uprights with your palms on top of the pins and facing each other.

Movement Performance
With your hands locked in place around the upright and resting on top of the pins, allow your feet to slowly come off the floor and at the same time hold your grip firmly around the posts.

The starting position will be hands above the head in a wide V shape, with your feet curled up enough to keep from touching the floor. Slowly pull yourself up and somewhat back, to the point where your ears are at eye level. Slowly lower yourself back to the starting point and repeat for the desired number of reps.

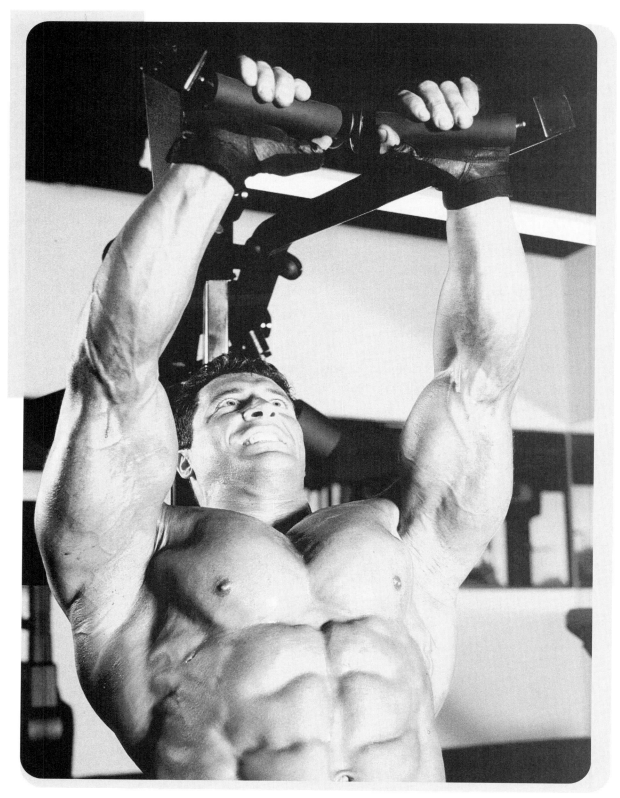

Milos Sarcev

3

CHEST TRAINING

MUSCLES OF THE CHEST

The muscles that bodybuilders call the chest group are the pectoralis major, pectoralis minor, and the subclavius. The largest of the group are the **pectoralis major** muscles. These are the large, thick, fan-shaped muscles of the upper chest wall that act on the joint of the shoulder. The pectoralis major serves to flex, adduct, and medially rotate the arm in the shoulder joint.

The **pectoralis minor** are thin, triangular muscles of the upper chest wall beneath the pectoralis major. They function to rotate the scapula, to draw it down and forward. The **subclavius** is a short, cylindrical muscle of the chest wall. The subclavius acts to draw the shoulder down and forward.

The pectoral muscles contract to pull the humerus from a position with the elbow well behind the body to one in which the elbow is forward and well across the midline of the body. By pulling your arm across your body at various points you can selectively stress different parts of your pec muscles. For example, pulling your arm across your torso below shoulder level stresses the lower portion of the pecs; pulling it across at shoulder level stresses the lower portion of the pecs; and pulling it across your torso above shoulder level places greater stress on your upper pecs.

GENERAL CHEST TRAINING POINTERS

Getting dumbbells off the floor and into the correct starting position to perform any type of Dumbbell Press or Flye can be a chore and the ultimate joint wrecker.

For flat benches, assume a position at one end of a heavy-duty bench and rest dumbbells on end against the tops of your thighs. Keeping your legs flexed toward your torso, roll backward onto the bench with your arms straight. This will bring the dumbbells to arm's length. To return to the starting point, you simply draw or curl up your legs placing your lower thighs against the ends of the dumbbells, and roll forward into an upright position.

The technique for incline dumbbell work is to assume the same position on an incline bench as in Flat Flyes and Presses. The dumbbells are then lifted one at a time by lifting one knee at a time to a point where the dumbbell is resting at shoulder level. Then repeat for the other arm.

In the decline use of dumbbells, you roll back from the initial starting point as in Flat Flyes and Presses—you should have a training partner or spotter stand at either side. When you have completed the rep goal, they can then simply grasp the appropriate weight at either end very firmly.

Now let's launch a total chest assault plan with three steps.

1. Read through the 19 chest exercises on the following pages.
2. Select 3 or 4 different exercises based on your goals.
3. Get busy training chest and never look back.

Bench Press

Muscles Involved
This exercise is responsible for the tremendous degree of chest development seen in today's champions. Bench Presses are considered to be one of the best exercises for the upper body. Bench Presses stress the pectoralis major and minor, deltoids, and triceps brachia. Secondary emphasis is on the latissimus dorsi.

Position

Load the bar on the bench with collars on each end of the bar. Lie back on the bench with your shoulders about 3–4 inches toward the foot end of the bench from the rack supports.

Place your feet on the floor to balance your body on the bench as you do the movement. Take an overgrip on the bar with your hands set about 2–4 inches past shoulder width.

Your forearms should be straight up and down in relation to the floor at all times during the exercise. If your hand spacing is too wide, then excessive stress is thrust onto the shoulder joint.

Movement Performance

Straighten your arms to remove the barbell from the rack and move it to a supported position directly above your shoulder joints.

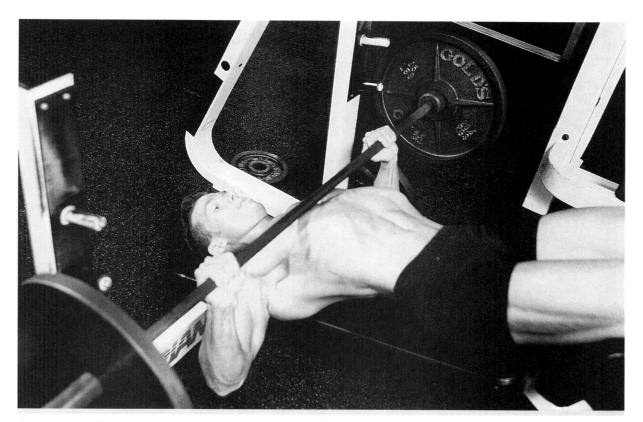

Bench Press Jonathan Lawson

Making sure that your elbows travel directly out to the sides, bend your arms and slowly lower the barbell from the supported position downward to the bottom of your pectoral muscles.

Touch the bar to your chest for only a split second. Without bouncing the weight, slowly push it back to straight arm's length. Repeat the movement until you complete the correct number of reps.

Tips

The most common variation in this movement is moving your grip inward or outward. When you use a grip of less than shoulder width, you shift the stress more to the inner pectorals and triceps.

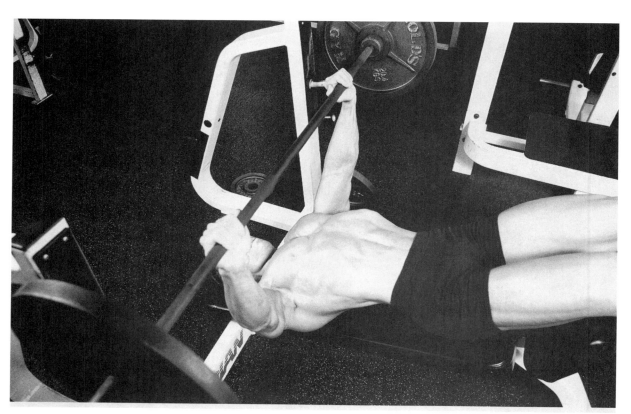

Bench Press Jonathan Lawson

A wider than normal grip places more stress onto the outer pectorals and anterior deltoids. In addition to changing your grip, there are a number of other very effective twists on a conventional Bench Press.

An extra level of controlled smoothness and safety is provided by the Smith Machine Bench, on which the training technique is essentially the same as for conventional bench presses. Pay attention to the position of the safety catches on the Smith when you train alone.

Machine Bench Press

Muscles Involved
This exercise works the pectoralis major and minor, deltoids, and triceps brachia muscles. Secondary emphasis is on the latissimus dorsi.

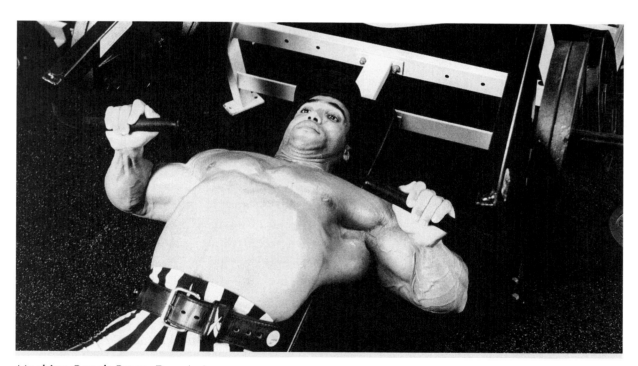

Machine Bench Press Dennis James

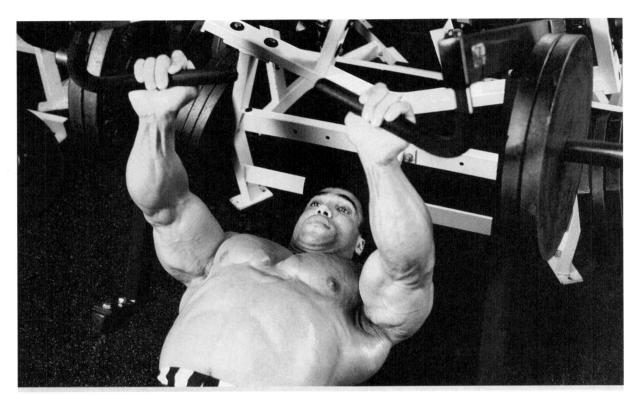

Machine Bench Press   Dennis James

Position

Adjust the seat to the appropriate position for your height. You are able to train with heavier than normal weights on a Machine Bench Press because of the added leverage and a decreased need for secondary muscle stabilization. Load the plates or select the resistance accordingly.

Sit or lie back in a position where the bar or handles are in line with the bottom section of your chest. Place your feet solidly on the floor. Place your hands in a grip set about 2–4 inches past shoulder width.

Movement Performance

From the bottom position, straighten your arms to directly above your shoulder joints. Push up on the handles or bar and straighten your arms to a point just before a complete lockout.

Squeeze your pectorals together at the top and then begin the eccentric motion. Making sure that your elbows move directly out to the sides, bend your arms and slowly lower the resistance to the bottom starting point.

Dumbbell Bench Press

Muscles Involved
Dumbbell Bench Presses stress the upper area of the pectoralis major and minor, deltoids, and triceps brachii muscles. Secondary emphasis is on the latissimus dorsi.

Position
Grasp two appropriately heavy dumbbells and lie back on the bench. Hold the dumbbells at approximately shoulder width. Bring the weights to straight arm's length directly above your shoulder joints and rotate your wrists so that your palms are facing toward the ceiling as with a regular barbell.

Movement Performance
Being careful that your upper arms move directly out to the sides, slowly lower the dumbbells to where they are in line with the side of your torso at slightly below the top of your chest.

At the bottom level your elbows should be slightly below the level of your torso. From this bottom stretch, return the dumbbells back along the same line of travel to the starting point. Repeat for the targeted rep count.

Incline Press

Muscles Involved
Incline Presses, whether performed with a barbell, two dumbbells, or on a machine, all train pectoralis major and minor, deltoids, and triceps brachii. Secondary emphasis is on the latissimus dorsi. One difference between performing presses on the inclines

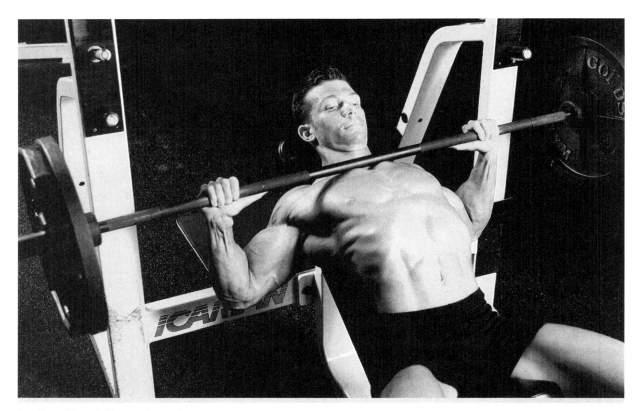

Incline Bench Press Jonathan Lawson

and flat benches is that using the incline shifts an increased work-load onto the anterior section of the deltoids.

Position
Place a barbell on the upright support racks of an incline bench. Load the weight on the bar and use collars on each end. Sit down on the bench's seat and lie back with your feet tucked slightly underneath your hips.

Maintain a slight arch in your lower back and keep your feet firmly on the floor. Take an over-grip on the bar with your hands set 3–5 inches wider than shoulder width. Straighten your arms to remove the barbell from the rack and bring it to a supported position directly above your shoulder joints.

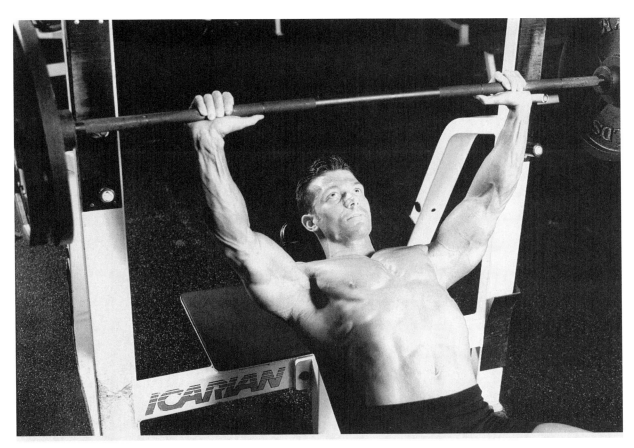

Incline Bench Press Jonathan Lawson

Movement Performance
Keeping your elbows back, slowly bend your arms and lower the barbell down to lightly touch your upper chest at the base of your neck. Without bouncing the bar off your chest, steadily push the barbell back to the starting point. Repeat for desired number of reps.

Tips
As with Bench Presses, you can vary the width of your grip when performing Incline Barbell Presses. You may also use any number of different angles with adjustable incline benches.

Machine Iso-Incline Press

Muscles Involved

If you are after even further upper chest size than you can attain
by doing Incline Barbell Presses, give the machine version a try.
As in the conventional barbell movement the pectoralis major and
minor, deltoids, and triceps brachii muscles all receive the brunt
of the workload. Secondary emphasis is on the latissimus dorsi.

Position

Adjust the seat to the appropriate position for your height. Load
the plates or select the resistance. Sit or lie back in a position

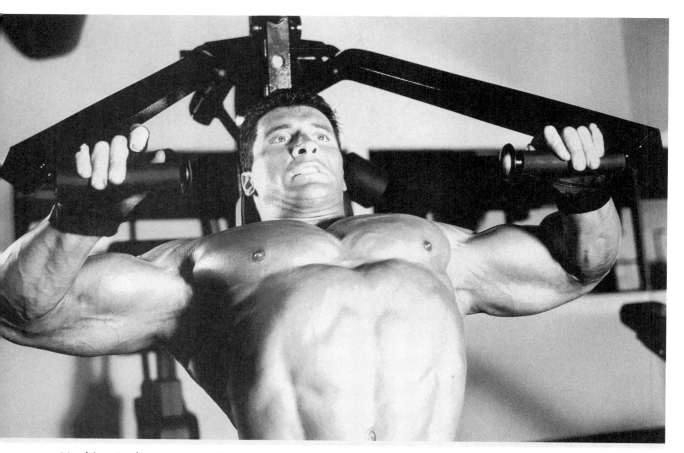

Machine Incline Press Milos Sarcev

where the handles are in line with the bottom section of your chest. Place your feet solidly on the floor. Place your hands in a grip set about 2–4 inches past shoulder width.

Movement Performance
From the bottom position, straighten your arms to directly above your shoulder joints. As you move past the midpoint of the motion, the handles should simultaneously be drawn together to a point where the handles are nearly touching.

Tightly squeeze your pectorals together at the top and then begin the eccentric motion downward. Being careful that your elbows move directly out to the sides, bend your arms and slowly lower the resistance to the bottom starting point.

Tip
As opposed to conventional Barbell Inclines, Machine Inclines provide an isolateral movement. This individual axis of rotation allows each arm to move independently of one another. In many aspects this exercise is similar to Dumbbell Inclines.

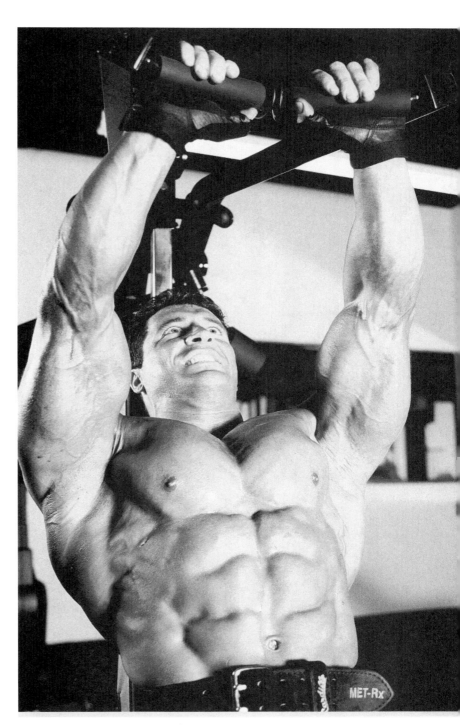

Machine Incline Press Milos Sarcev

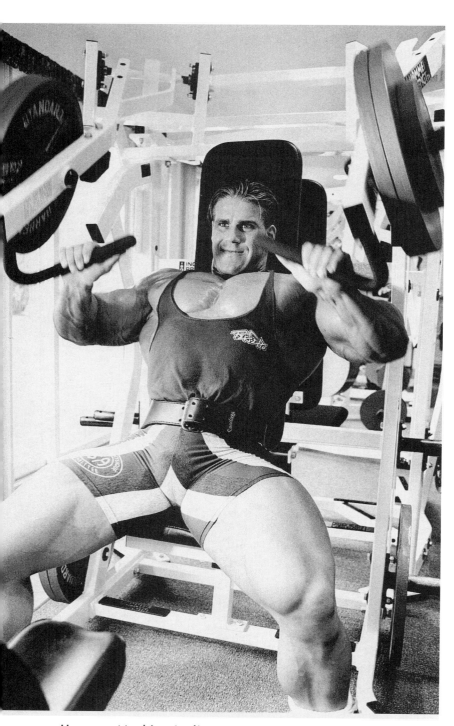

Hammer Machine Incline Press Jay Cutler

Hammer Machine Incline Press

Muscles Involved
As in the other types of Machine Incline, Hammer Inclines work the upper pectoralis major and minor, deltoids, and triceps brachii muscles. Secondary emphasis is on the latissimus dorsi.

Position
Adjust the seat to the appropriate position for your height. Load the plates. Lie back in a position where the handles are in line with the bottom section of your chest. Place your feet solidly on the floor. Place your hands in a grip set about 2–4 inches past shoulder width.

Movement Performance
Straighten your arms to a point just before a complete lockout. Squeeze your pectorals together at the top and then begin the eccentric motion. Making sure that your elbows move directly out to the sides, bend your arms and slowly lower the resistance to the bottom starting point. Repeat for the desired number of reps.

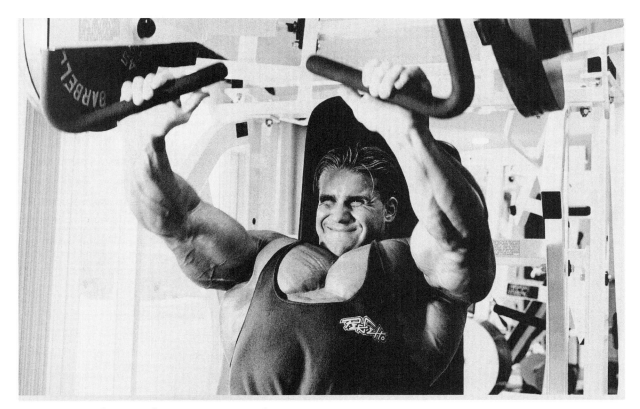

Hammer Machine Incline Press Jay Cutler

Tip
This machine also is produced in a dual-axis arrangement in
which the handles do not move independently of one another.

Dumbbell Incline Bench Press

Muscles Involved
Incline Presses performed with dumbbells train the upper pectoralis major and minor, deltoids, and triceps brachii muscles.
Secondary emphasis is on the latissimus dorsi. As the angle of the
bench approaches parallel to the floor, more of the workload
shifts onto the lower pectorals. As the incline increases toward a
90-degree angle, then more of the workload shifts onto the upper
chest and shoulder area.

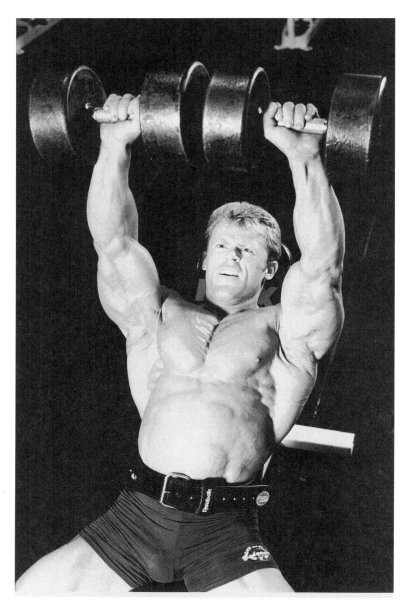

Dumbbell Incline Bench Press Art Dikes

Position

Grasp two appropriately heavy dumbbells and lie back on the bench. Bring the weights to straight arm's length directly above your head and shoulder joints. Rotate your wrists so that your palms are facing toward the ceiling as with a regular barbell. The dumbbells should be held at approximately shoulder width.

Movement Performance

Allowing the elbows to move out to your sides, slowly lower the dumbbells to where they are in line with the side of your torso slightly below the top of your chest. At the bottom level your elbows should be slightly below the level of your torso. From this bottom stretch, return the dumbbells back along the same line of travel to the starting point. Repeat for the desired number of reps.

Tips

Use a different bench every so often; this will keep the chest development not only massive but correctly proportioned. If you have trouble making the adjustment from flat benches to inclines, then give some consideration to the Incline Machine Press. The angle change can be tough until you get the hang of it, and the machine movement provides the needed "groove."

Barbell Decline Bench Press

Muscles Involved
Decline Presses stimulate and stress your lower pectoralis major and minor, deltoids, and triceps brachii. Secondary emphasis is on the latissimus dorsi. The angle of the bench determines the amount of work performed by different areas of your pectorals. The higher your feet are in relation to your head, the greater the workload thrust upon the lower portion of your pecs.

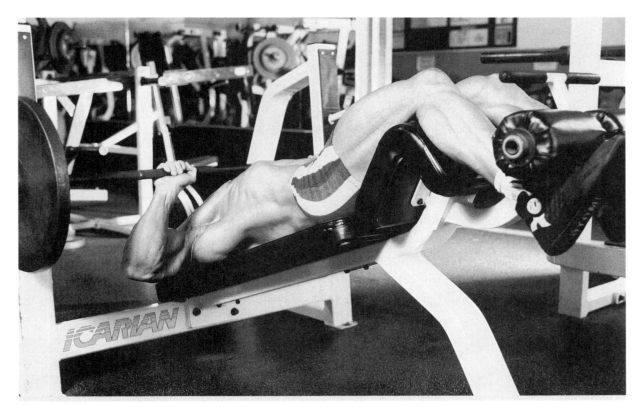

Barbell Decline Bench Press Remi Zuri

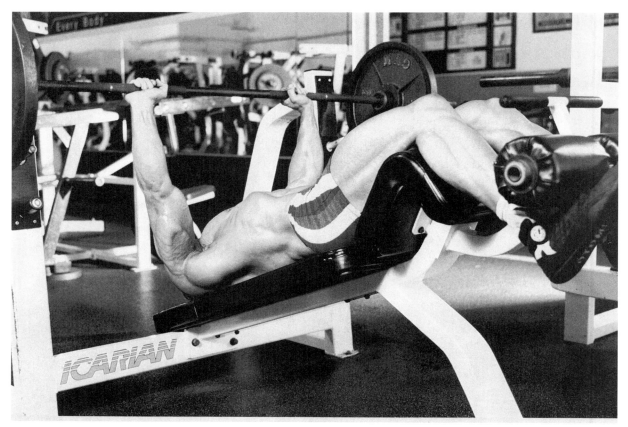

Barbell Decline Bench Press Remi Zuri

Position

Adjust the support racks on the decline bench so that you will be able to smoothly return the bar to the rack upon completion of the movement. Rest a barbell loaded to the appropriate weight on the supports using a collar on each end. Sit down on the end opposite the support racks and hook your feet under the restraining bar.

Carefully lie back and slip your head under the bar, arching your lower back. Take an over-grip on the bar with your hands 3–5 inches wider than shoulder width. Straighten your arms to lift the bar off the racks and directly over the line of your shoulder joints.

Movement Performance
Keeping your elbows back, slowly bend your arms and lower the barbell down to touch the lower part of your chest at your pec line. Without any bouncing, slowly push the weight back to straight arm's length. Repeat the movement for the desired repetition count.

Dumbbell Decline Bench Press

Muscles Involved
Dumbbell Decline Presses stimulate and stress your lower pectoralis major and minor, deltoids, and triceps brachii. Secondary emphasis is on the latissimus dorsi.

Position
Grasp two appropriately heavy dumbbells and sit back on top of the padded knee rest. As you begin to lay backwards onto the bench, carefully rock the dumbbells up and onto the lower portion of your chest.

Press the dumbbells to arm's length directly above your shoulder joints and rotate your wrists so that your palms are facing toward the ceiling as with a regular barbell. The dumbbells should be held at approximately shoulder width.

Movement Performance
Keeping your elbows underneath the dumbbells, slowly bend your arms and lower them to the lower, outside edge of your chest. From this bottom position, slowly push the dumbbells back to straight arm's length. Repeat for the desired number of reps.

Incline Dumbbell Flye

Muscles Involved
The advantage to including flyes in your chest training is their ability to isolate your triceps out of the movement and place

direct stress on your upper pectorals. Secondary stress is on your deltoids and triceps.

You can select the area of your pectorals that you wish to stress by the angle of the bench you pick to use for the exercise. When the bench is parallel to the floor there is slightly more workload onto the lower pectorals. As the incline increases toward a 90-degree angle, then the workload shifts onto the upper chest and shoulder area.

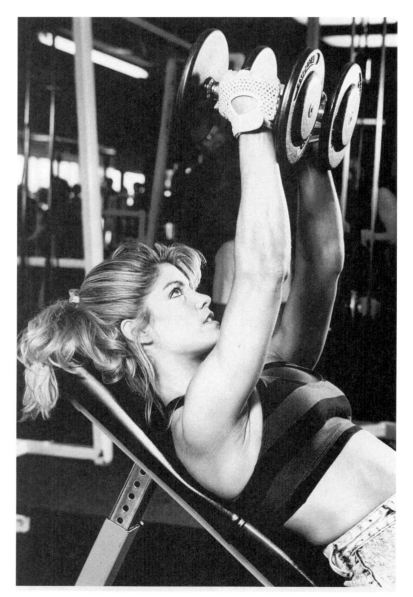

Incline Dumbbell Flye Dana Dodson

Position

Grab two appropriately heavy dumbbells and lean backward onto the bench. Carefully rock the dumbbells to the front of your shoulders as you lean back. Then press them to arm's length directly above your shoulder joints and rotate your wrists so that your palms are facing each other. Bend your arms about 10 degrees and maintain this slightly bent arm position throughout the movement.

Movement Performance

Being sure that your upper arms move directly out to the sides, slowly lower the dumbbells in semicircular arcs to a low but stretched position. At the bottom your elbows should be slightly below the level of your torso.

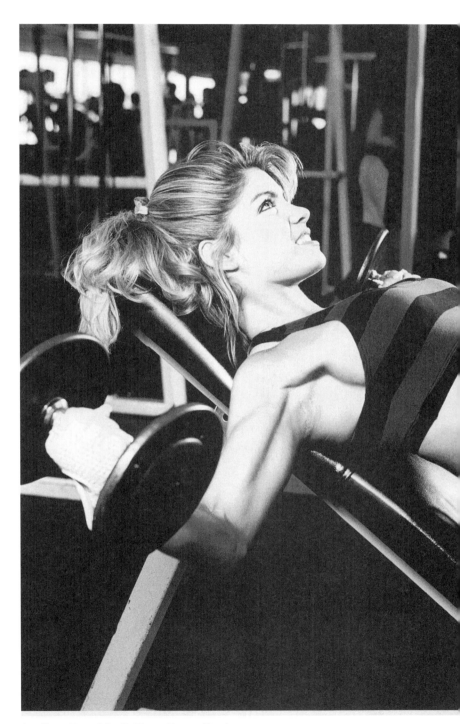

Using just the power of your chest, slowly return the weights back along the same arc of travel to the starting point. Make every attempt to squeeze your pectorals together as you reach the top position. Repeat for the desired number of reps.

Incline Cable Flye

Muscles Involved
When you perform Incline Flyes with cables, you shift the muscular balance as compared to Incline Flyes with dumbbells. This is due to the angle of the pulley relative to the weight. The pectoralis major and minor, deltoids, triceps brachii, and latissimus dorsi muscles are all involved in this movement.

Position
Position the incline bench so that the upper end of the bench is in line with the pulleys. Be certain to center the bench halfway between the weight stacks. Sit down on the bench and with your right hand pick up the right pulley. Sit upright and repeat this process with your left hand.

Incline Dumbbell Flye Dana Dodson

With pulleys in hand, lean back while at the same time bringing the handles to shoulder height. Press the back of your shoulders against the bench for support.

From shoulder height, simultaneously press the handles to an overhead position. Rotate your wrists so that your palms are facing each other. Bend your arms about 10 degrees and maintain this rounded-arm position throughout the movement.

Movement Performance

Being sure that your upper arms travel directly out to the sides, slowly lower the handles, keeping them under control at all times. Follow a semicircular path, ending in a low but comfortably stretched position. It is important to keep your hands steady throughout the entire range of the motion.

From the bottom of the movement at the moment of maximum stretch, push back up on the handles using your forearms as pistons, and reverse the movement back up to the starting point. Increase the intensity of your contraction as you pass the halfway point, reaching a maximum at the completion of the repetition. Repeat for the desired number of reps.

Machine Flye

Muscles Involved

This exercise is similar to the Pec Dec in many respects. When performing Pec Decs you use your forearms to push against the pads to lift the weight. In the case of Machine Flyes the hands are used to move the weight.

Machine Flye equipment is generally designed as a flat bench or an incline bench. This exercise allows you to isolate most of the stress on the pectoralis major and minor, with secondary involvement of your deltoids.

Position

For Flat Bench Machine Flyes, assume a position on the bench that aligns your lower pectoral area with the handles. Bring the handles up from their resting position and center them over your mid-pectoral.

In the case of Incline Machine Flyes, adjust the seat to a height that puts your upper chest in line with the handles. Sit on the seat, facing away from the weight stack. With your palms facing together, grab the handles so that your shoulders are just slightly ($\frac{1}{2}$–1 inch) above a line formed by your pectorals, elbows, and the handles. In order to start this exercise you first must lift (or have a spotter help lift) the weight into the starting position.

Movement Performance
Allowing a slight bend at the elbow, push tighter until the handles touch in front of your face. Keep the elbows at the same angle through the entire range of motion. Tightly squeeze your pectorals together as the handles touch.

Then, continuing to hold the elbows at the level of the handles, begin to reverse the motion back to the bottom position. Hold constant tension on the weight at all times, especially during the lowering portion. Carefully reach a maximum stretch at the bottom. Then continue for the rest of your repetitions.

Flat Bench Dumbbell Flye

Muscles Involved
When you perform Flat Bench Dumbbell Flyes, you effectively remove your triceps from the exercise. This results in isolation for the pectoralis major and minor, deltoids, and triceps brachii. Secondary emphasis is on the latissimus dorsi. When the bench is parallel to the floor, more work is demanded from your lower pectorals.

Position
Grab two appropriately heavy dumbbells and lie back onto the bench. Carefully rock the dumbbells to the front of your shoulders as you lean back. Then press them to arm's length directly above your shoulder joints. Rotate your wrists so that your palms are fac-

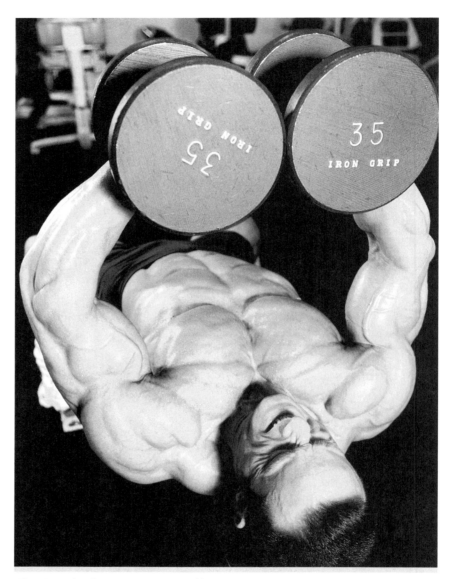

Flat Bench Flye Porter Cottrell

ing each other. Bend your arms about 10 degrees and maintain this slightly bent arm position throughout the movement.

Movement Performance
Being careful that your upper arms move directly out to the sides, slowly lower the dumbbells in semicircular arcs to a low but

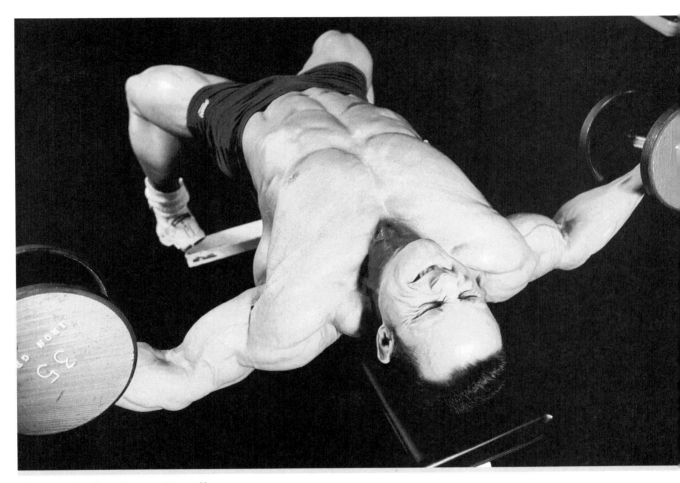

Flat Bench Flye Porter Cottrell

stretched position. At the bottom level your elbows should be
slightly below the level of your torso.

As you see in the accompanying photos, it is essential to
safely yet completely stretch the chest. In a sense you can visual-
ize the edges of your torso being drawn down and over the lower
edge of the bench. Using your mind to see yourself performing
your flyes will allow for complete expansion of the upper torso.

Using just the power of your chest, slowly return the weights
back along the same arc of travel to the starting point. Make
every attempt to squeeze your pectorals together as you reach the
top position.

Flat Bench Cable Flye

Muscles Involved
When you perform Flat Bench Flyes with cables, you shift the muscular balance as compared to Flat Bench Flyes with dumbbells. This is due to the angle of the pulley relative to the weight. Your pectoralis major and minor are isolated in this exercise. Less work is performed by the deltoids, triceps, and latissimus dorsi.

Position
Center a flat bench between the cable uprights. Attach a handle to the end of each cable and lay the cables at right angles to the bench. Sit down at the end of the bench furthest from the handles.

Lay back on the bench and firmly plant your feet on the floor. Slightly tilt your upper body to the right and with your right hand grab the cable handle. Bring the handle to the middle of your chest. Next, repeat this process for the left side.

Movement Performance
Press the handles to an overhead position. The palms of your hands should be facing toward each other during the entire exercise. Slowly begin to allow the handles to move downward with your arms slightly bent at the elbows.

During the first half of the motion keep your forearms at right angles (90 degrees) to the floor. As your elbows break the plane of the bench, the angle of your forearm shifts to one of 45 degrees relative to the floor.

Decline Bench Dumbbell Flye

Muscles Involved
When you perform flyes, you can isolate your triceps from the movement and place very direct stress on your lower pecs and

anterior deltoids. Secondary stress is on your medial deltoids and triceps. You can select the area of your pectorals that you wish to stress by the angle of the bench you pick to use for the exercise.

Position
Grasp two appropriately heavy dumbbells and lie back on the particular bench chosen. Bring the weights to straight arm's length directly above your shoulder joints and rotate your wrists so that your palms are facing each other. Bend your arms about 10 degrees and maintain this rounded-arm position throughout the movement.

Movement Performance
Being sure that your upper arms move directly out to the sides, slowly lower the dumbbells in semicircular arcs to a low but comfortably stretched position. At the bottom level your elbows should be slightly below the level of your torso.

Using just the power of your chest, slowly return the weights back along the same arc of travel to the starting point. Repeat for the targeted rep count.

Cable Crossover

Muscles Involved
This exercise typifies the exercises known as "cutting or refining movements." This is due to the tremendous pectoral isolation that is inherent in this type of movement. You cannot use "heavy weights" when doing Cable Crossovers, so to achieve superior results it is essential to use only the pectoral strength when you perform this exercise.

Cable Crossovers work primarily the pectoralis major and minor and the deltoids. Crossovers are frequently used to razor in deep grooves across the chest before contests.

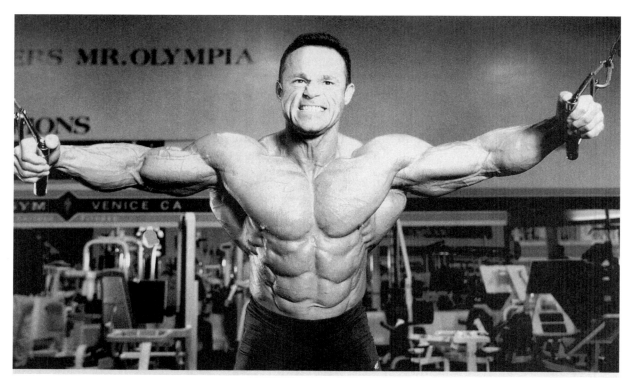

Cable Crossover Porter Cottrell

Position

Attach loop handles to the cables running through high pulleys. Stand between the pulleys with your feet set about shoulder width apart and grasp the two pulley handles.

With your palms down throughout the movement, extend your arms upward at about a 45-degree angle in relation to the floor. Bend your arms slightly during the exercise.

Movement Performance

Use pectoral strength to move your hands downward in semicircular arcs and toward each other until they touch 6–8 inches in front of your hips.

Hold this position for a brief second. Then allow your hands to slowly return to the starting point and repeat for the desired number of reps.

Tip
Normally, your torso will be
either erect or inclined
slightly forward during this
exercise.

Parallel Bar Dip

Muscles Involved
This is an excellent upper
body movement that stresses
the pectoralis major and
minor, deltoids, and triceps
brachii muscles with phenomenal intensity. Due to the total
upper body involvement with
any type of dip, the latissimus
dorsi receive their share of the
work. The pectoralis emphasis
is primarily on the lower and
outer sections of the pecs.

Position
There are two different types
of dipping bars. The first is a
V-shaped design; the second
design is built with the bars
running parallel to each
other. Regardless of the bars
used, take a grip that will
have your palms facing
toward each other. Step up
and straighten your arms.

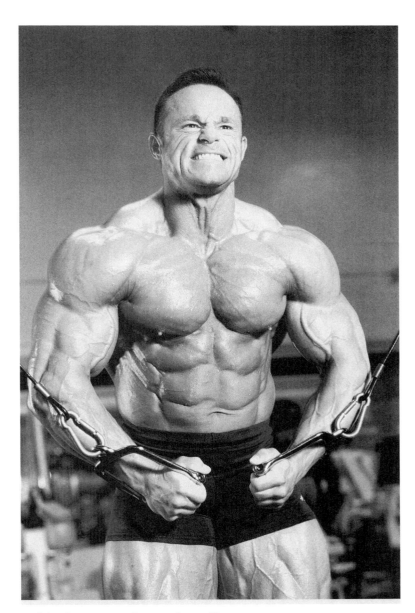

Cable Crossover Porter Cottrell

For the exact starting position, hold your body at arm's
length above the bars and bend your legs slightly for upper body
stability. Lower your chin and incline your upper body forward.

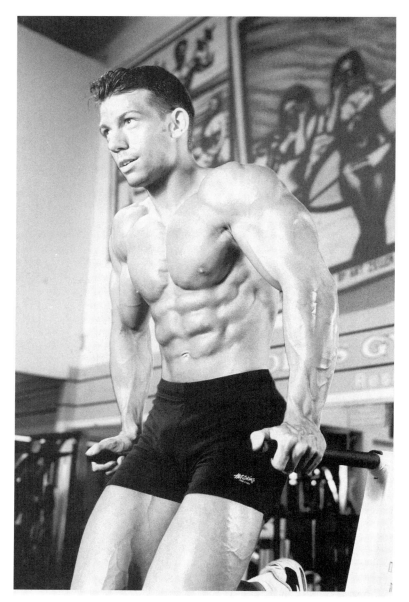

Dip Jonathan Lawson

Note: For more triceps development, perform your dips with the torso at a 90-degree angle to the floor without any tipping forward of the torso.

Movement Performance
Allowing your elbows to move out to the sides, bend your arms and slowly lower yourself as far below the bars as possible. From the bottom point, slowly push yourself back up until your arms are straight. Repeat for the required repetition count.

As illustrated in the second dipping photo, there is an outrageously intense stretch felt across the entire pectoralis region. In this particular photo the two different pectoralis muscles are clearly delineated.

Tip
In the early stages of training, many novice bodybuilders find that they are not strong enough to effectively perform even as few as five repetitions of the dip. Often this exercise is simply too difficult to perform due to bodyweight versus strength issues.

As a solution to accommodate all levels of strength, Cybex has developed an assisted or self-spotting dip machine. This equipment provides a foot platform to stand on while performing the exercise. Instead of adding to the resistance, the foot platform acts as an adjustable counterbalance to your bodyweight. Some dipping machines have either a cable and waist belt attachment or foot platform incorporated into their actual design.

More advanced trainers can perform too many dips with their bodyweight and the problem here is one of adding to the level of resistance. Nautilus pioneered the use of a padded weight belt linked to an adjustable source of increased resistance. Even more elemental but also very effective is simply attaching a dumbbell to your lifting belt for more intensity.

Machine Dip

Muscles Involved
This is an excellent upper body movement that stresses the pectoralis major and minor, anterior deltoids, and

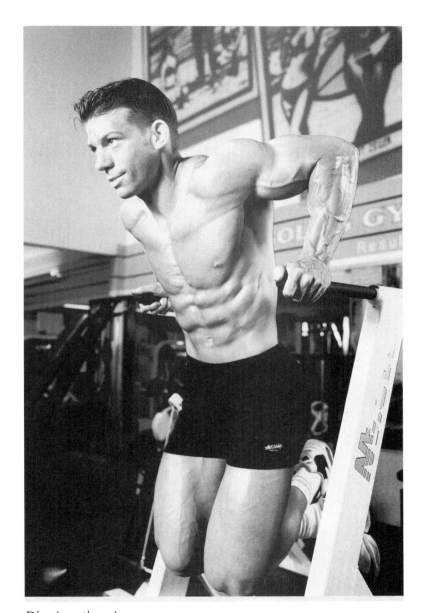

Dip Jonathan Lawson

triceps muscles with incredible intensity. The pectoralis emphasis is primarily on the lower and outer sections of the pecs. Secondary emphasis is on the medial deltoids and the upper back muscles responsible for rotating the scapulae.

Position
Take a grip that will have your palms facing toward each other, and then jump up to support your body at arm's length above the bars. Bend your legs for body stability, place your chin on your chest, and incline your torso forward.

Note: For more triceps development, perform your dips with the torso at a 90-degree angle to the floor without any tipping forward of the torso.

Movement Performance
Allowing your elbows to move out to the sides, bend your arms and slowly lower yourself as far below the bars as possible. From the bottom point, slowly push yourself back up until your arms are straight. Repeat for the required rep count.

Pec Dec

Muscles Involved
This movement allows you to isolate stress on your pecs with only minimal involvement of the anterior deltoids. You'll find this movement particularly good for adding mass to the inner edges of the pectorals where they originate from the sternum.

Position
Adjust the seat to a height that puts your upper arms parallel to the floor when you are sitting in the seat and allows your hands to rest over the top edge of the pads.

Sit on the seat facing away from the weight stack and place your elbows against the padded surface, your forearms running straight up the pads and your fingers curled over the top of the pads. Allow the weight to pull your elbows pads as far as comfortably possible to the rear.

Movement Performance
Use pec strength to push with your elbows against the pads, moving the pads forward until they touch each other directly in front

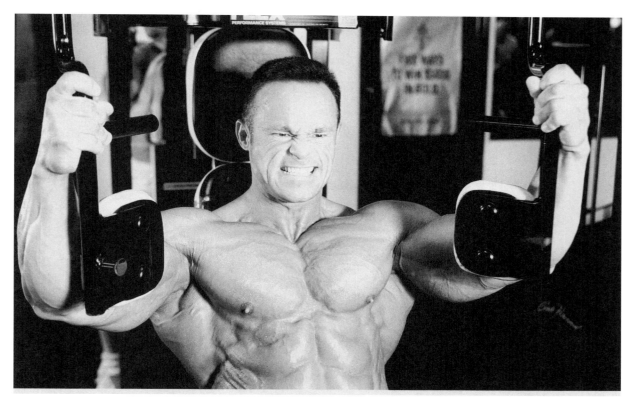

Pec Dec Machine Porter Cottrell

of you. Hold this peak position for a split second, and then allow the pads to slowly pull your elbows back to the initial starting point. Repeat for the correct rep count.

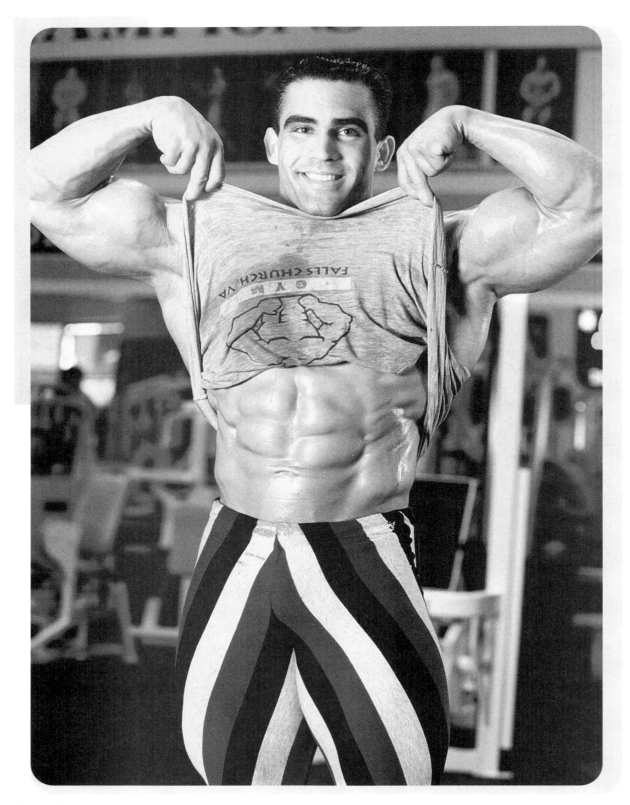

Abbas Katami

ABDOMINAL TRAINING

MUSCLES OF THE ABDOMEN

There are three muscle groups in the abdominals. The first of these is the **rectus abdominis**, the wall of muscle that covers the front of the abdomen and gives your abs a washboard appearance. Rectus abdominis are pairs of anterolateral muscles of the abdomen. Each pair extends the length of the abdomen. The muscles of each pair are separated by the linea alba. The rectus abdominis function to flex the vertebral column and to tense the anterior abdominal wall.

Also included in the discussion of frontal abdominals are the **pyramidalis**. The pyramidalis are anterolateral muscles of the abdomen that are contained in the lower end of the sheath of the rectus abdominis. They are small, triangular muscles that function to tense the linea alba.

The second important muscle group is the **obliques** at the sides of the hips. This group is usually called the external obliques, although there are really three layers of muscle there including the external, internal, and transversus abdominus muscles.

The **obliquus externus abdominis** are a pair of muscles that are the largest and the most superficial of the five anterolateral muscles of the abdomen. One side alone functions to bend the vertebral column laterally and to rotate it, drawing the shoulder of the same side forward.

The **obliquus internus abdominis** are a pair of anterolateral muscles of the abdomen that lie under the obliquus externus abdominis in the lateral and ventral part of the abdominal wall. These muscles are smaller and thinner than the obliquus externus abdominis. Both sides act together to flex the vertebral column. One side acting alone acts to bend the vertebral column laterally and rotate it, drawing the shoulder of the opposite side downward.

The **transversus abdominis** are a pair of transverse abdominal muscles that are the anterolateral muscles of the abdomen and lie immediately under the obliquus internus abdominis. They serve to constrict the abdomen.

The final muscle group includes the serratus anterior and the intercostals. The **serratus anterior** is a thin muscle of the chest wall extending from the ribs under the arm to the scapula. The serratus assists in the rotation of the scapula and the raising of the shoulder. The **intercostals** are the muscles between adjacent ribs. They are designated as external and internal, and function as breathing muscles.

Bench Leg Raise

Muscles Involved
All leg raise movements stress the entire abdominal area which includes the obliquus externus abdominis, obliquus internus abdominis, pyramidalis, rectus abdominis, and transversus abdominis muscles. In particular, the lower sections of the rectus abdominis are isolated.

Position
Bench Leg Raises are performed on a flat bench while holding the sides of the bench. As compared to leg raises on the floor, the advantage to Bench Leg Raises is that you can lower your feet

below the level of the rest of your body to increase the range of motion.

Place your hands on the edges of the bench to secure your body in position as you do the exercise. Bend your legs slightly and keep them bent throughout your set in order to keep undue stress off your lower back. You may perform this exercise with your feet crossed or held together.

Movement Performance
Use abdominal strength to move your feet in a semicircular arc from just below the level of the bench to just below the level of

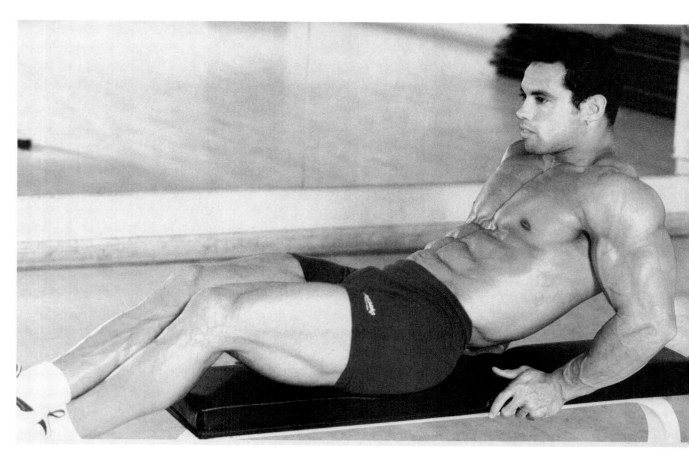

Bench Leg Raise Tito Raymond

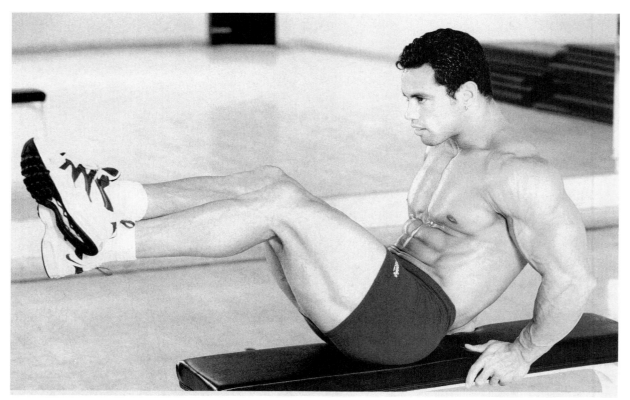

Bench Leg Raise Tito Raymond

your chin. The key to continuous tension is raising your legs only up to the point where your thighs are at a 45-degree angle with the floor. Return your feet slowly back to the starting point and repeat for the desired reps.

Floor Leg Raise

Muscles Involved
All leg raise movements stress the entire abdominal area which includes the obliquus externus abdominis, obliquus internus abdominis, pyramidalis, rectus abdominis, and transversus abdominis muscles. In particular, the lower sections of the rectus abdominis are isolated.

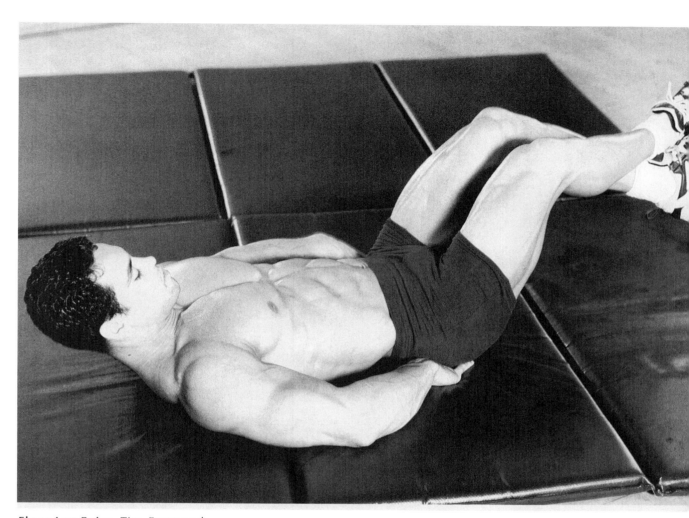

Floor Leg Raise Tito Raymond

Starting Position

Lie on your back on the floor. Place your hands underneath your glutes. Your forefingers and thumbs should form a triangle, palms down on the floor. Raise your head about two inches from the floor. Bend your legs slightly less than a 90-degree angle and draw your feet upward until they are 12 inches off the floor. Keep your legs in this position throughout your set in order to keep undue stress off your lower back.

Movement Performance
Use abdominal strength to move your feet in a semicircular arc from 12 inches off the floor to a point directly above your hips. Return your feet slowly back to the starting point and repeat for the desired reps.

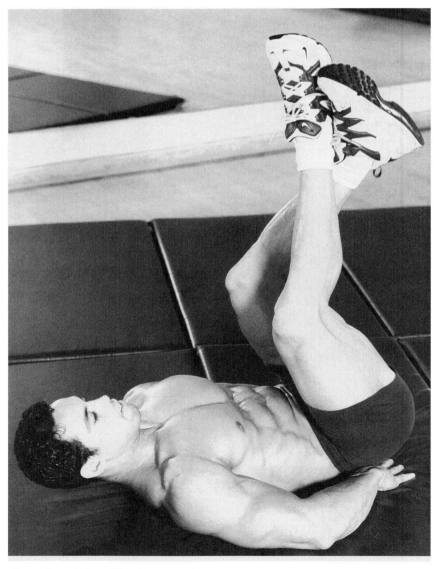

Floor Leg Raise Tito Raymond

Jack-Knife

Muscles Involved
This challenging movement stresses the entire abdominal area, including the obliquus externus abdominis, obliquus internus abdominis, pyramidalis, rectus abdominis, and transversus abdominis muscles.

Starting Position
Lie on your back on the floor. Place your hands above your head, thumbs together, palms up. Raise your feet up from the floor until

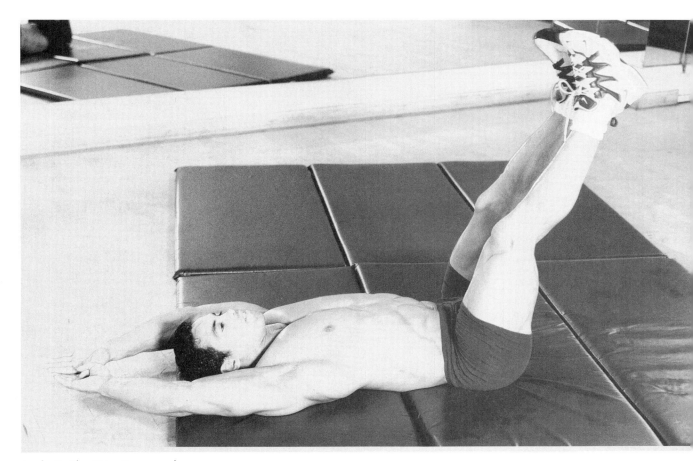

Jack-Knife Tito Raymond

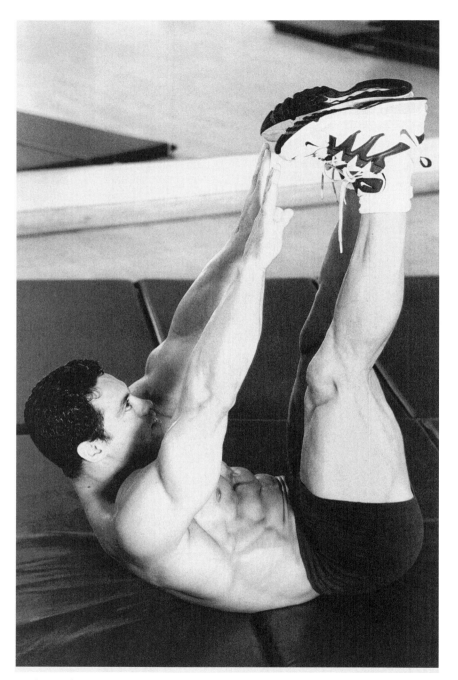

Jack-Knife Tito Raymond

your thighs are straight up and down. Bend your knees slightly so that your feet are in front of your knees. Keep your legs in this position throughout your set in order to keep undue stress off your lower back.

Movement Performance
Using abdominal strength only, move your arms and torso up off the floor until your hands touch your feet. Perform most of the movement with your upper body and not your legs. As your hands reach your feet, your upper back should be above the floor. The point of full contraction is when the hands and feet are directly above the navel. Return your upper back and arms slowly back to the starting point and repeat for the desired reps.

Side Crunch

Muscles Involved
This side abdominal area isolation movement is great for bringing out deep finger-like grooves in this area. Along with the side abdominals, this exercise also hits the rectus abdominis muscles.

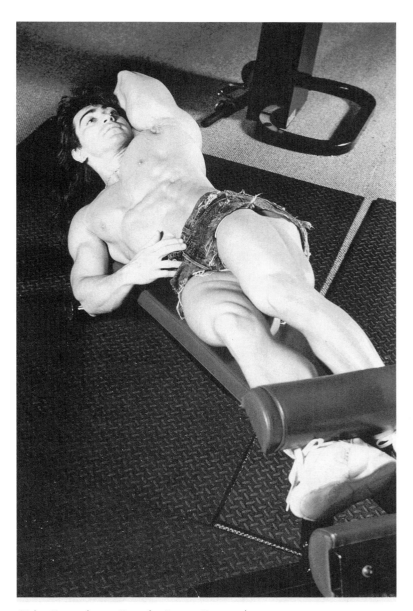

Side Crunch on Bench Steve Caropelo

Starting Position

Position an abdominal bench (with foot restraints) flat on the floor. Lay down on your right side so that when you hook your feet under the restraints, your feet are on their sides, pointed away from your torso. Tuck your left arm behind your head and lay your right on top of your navel. The correct starting position is with feet tucked under the restraints, right hip and shoulder against the bench, left hand tucked behind head, and right lying across the navel.

Movement Performance

The range of motion in this exercise is short. By intensely contracting your left abdominal area, draw your elbow toward your left hip. Your shoulders will only move a few inches. Move back and forth with full contraction. Repeat this short range of motion for the desired rep count. Switch sides and use the same position and movement for your right side.

Twisting Roman Chair Sit-Up

Muscles Involved
Roman Chair Sit-Ups stress the obliquus externus abdo-

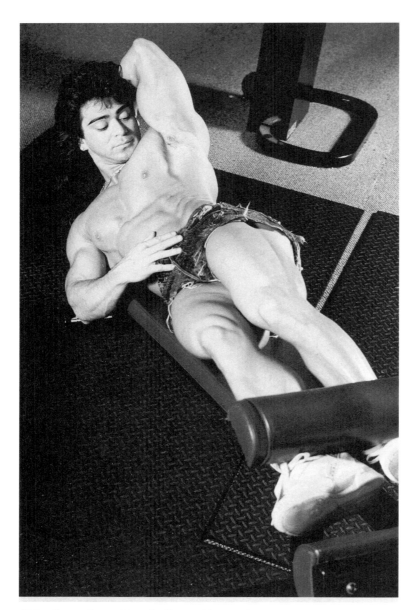

Side Crunch on Bench Steve Caropelo

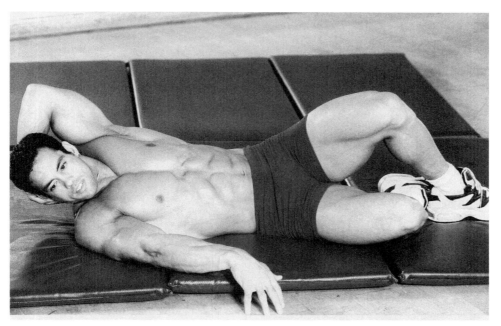

Side Crunch on Floor Tito Raymond

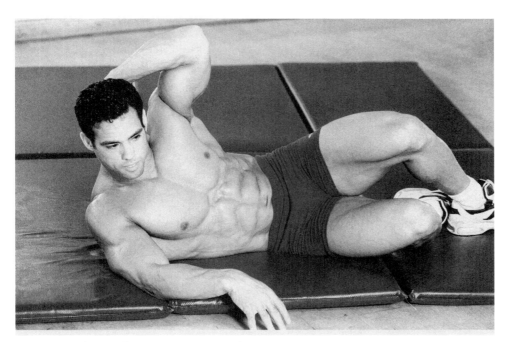

Side Crunch on Floor Tito Raymond

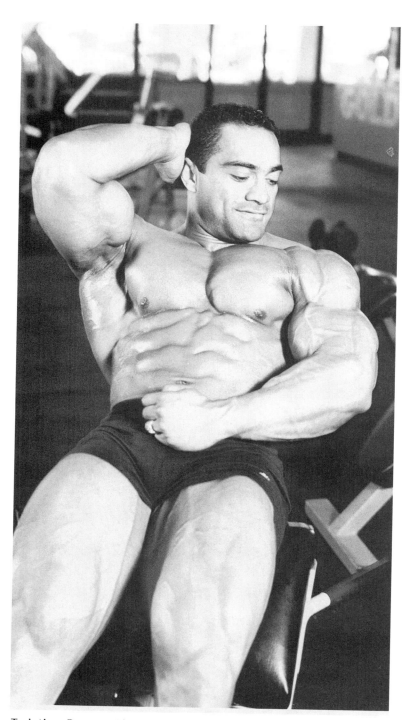

Twisting Roman Chair Sit-Up Tevita Aholelei

minis, obliquus internus abdominis, pyramidalis, rectus abdominis, and transversus abdominis muscles.

Position
Sit on the bench seat facing toward the toe restraint/wedge. Place the front portion of each foot under the pads. Place your right hand behind your head and your left just under the navel. Keep your hands and arms in this position throughout the movement. Turn your head to look across your left shoulder. Sit and move your torso backward to approximately a 30-degree angle to the floor.

Movement Performance
The range of motion in this exercise is short. By intensely contracting your right abdominal area, draw your right elbow towards your right hip. Your right shoulder will move only a few inches. Move back and forth with a full contraction. Repeat this short range of motion for the desired rep count. Switch to your left hand behind head and right hand on lower abdominals and repeat for your left side.

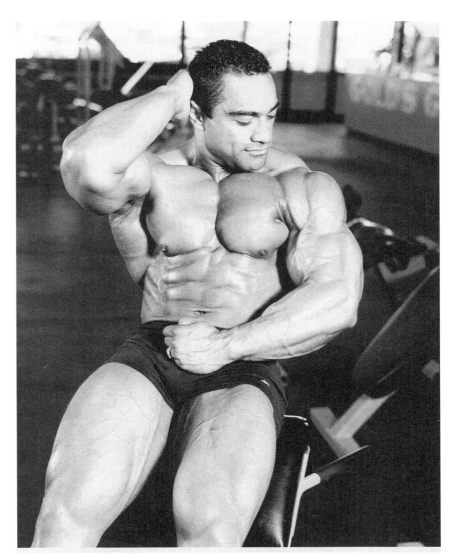

Twisting Roman Chair Sit-Up Tevita Aholelei

Rope and Cable Crunch

Muscles Involved
Rope and Cable Crunches burn their blowtorch cuts across the
entire abdominal area.

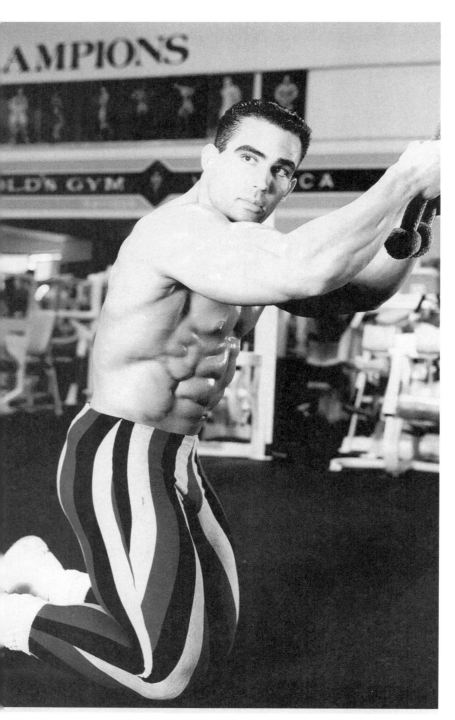

Rope and Cable Crunch Abbas Katami

Position
Attach a rope handle to an overhead cable and grasp the two ends of the rope extending down from the cable with your hands. Kneel down about a foot back from the weight stack and extend your body toward the pulley.

Movement Performance
You must simultaneously perform three tasks in order to do an effective Rope and Cable Crunch:

- Bend over at the waist until your forehead touches the floor.
- Do a small, pullover movement to bring your arms from an extended position to one in which they are bent at 90-degree angles and your hands are near the floor just ahead of your head.
- Forcefully exhale all of your air.

When you perform these three tasks, you will feel a strong contraction in your abs. Hold this contraction for a second, and then return to the starting point. Repeat for the desired rep count.

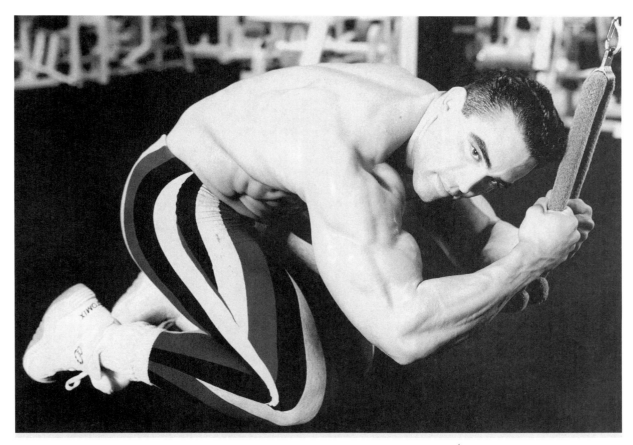

Rope and Cable Crunch Abbas Katami

Tip
This movement can be performed with one arm at a time, but be sure to keep the reps balanced on both sides.

Floor Crunch

Muscles Involved
Crunches of any type are one of the most direct exercises for stressing the abdominal wall. This includes the obliquus externus abdominis, obliquus internus abdominis, pyramidalis, rectus abdominis, and transversus abdominis muscles.

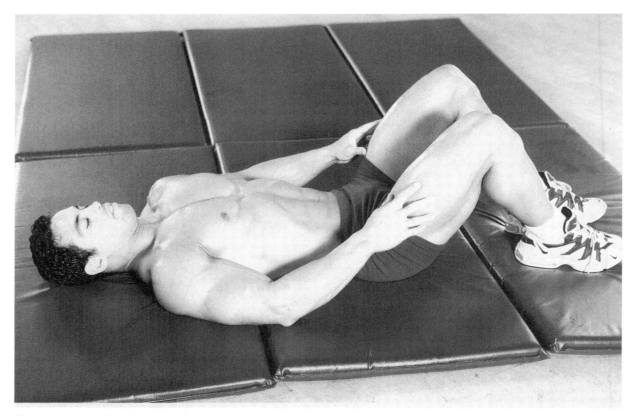

Floor Crunch Tito Raymond

Starting Position
Lie on your back on the floor with your legs bent at 90-degree angles and your feet flat on the floor. Place your hands on top of your thighs and your elbows on the floor next to your torso.

Movement Performance
You must do four things at once to perform this crunch:

- Force your shoulders toward your hips.
- Use lower abdominal strength to raise your hips from the floor.
- Use upper abdominal strength to raise your head and shoulders off the floor.
- Forcefully exhale your air.

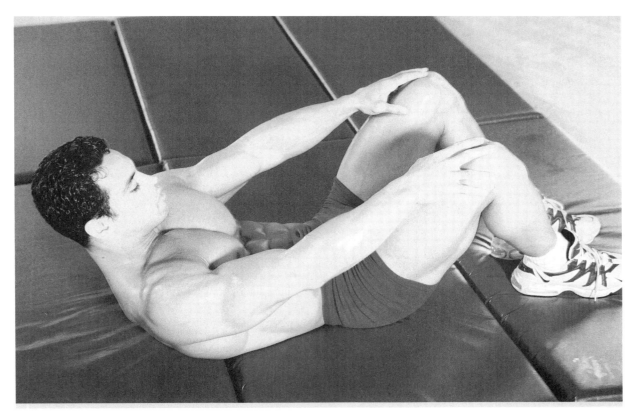

Floor Crunch Tito Raymond

When you perform these four tasks simultaneously, you will feel a very powerful contraction in your front abdominal wall. Hold this contraction for a brief moment, then lower yourself back to the starting point and repeat for the desired number of reps.

Tips

You can perform Wall Crunches in which you lie on the floor with your glutes in the corner formed by the floor and wall, and with your legs running straight up the wall. Or you can hold your knees at a 90-degree angle with your feet flat against the wall. A "one hand behind the head" twisting motion is a great way to inject some alternative stress across the side abdominal areas.

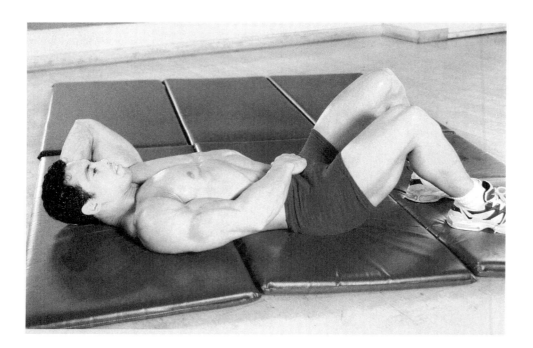

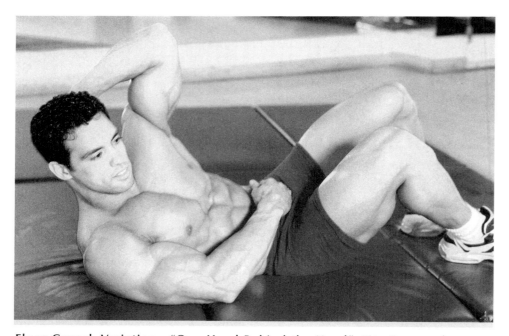

Floor Crunch Variation—"One Hand Behind the Head" Tito Raymond

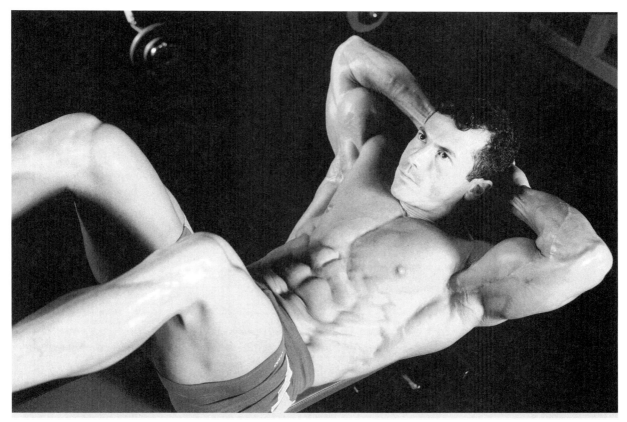

Floor Crunch with Knees at 90 Degrees B. J. Quinn

Machine Crunch

Muscles Involved
Machine Crunches provide a convenient method of adding resistance to the exercise.

Position
Sit on the seat and adjust according to your frame. Hook your feet under the restraints provided. Reach back and grasp the handles of the machine. Put your chin to your chest at the starting point of the movement.

Movement Performance
Perform the crunch movement as previously described, hold the
point of peak contraction for a second, then return to the starting
point and repeat for the desired number of reps.

Tip
Some machines have a set of upper chest area pads that you
place your chest against to provide a point of contact with the
machine. This is as opposed to grasping handles as detailed
above.

Reverse Crunch

Muscles Involved
Reverse Crunches place tremendous stress on all members of the
abdominal groups: the obliquus externus abdominis, obliquus
internus abdominis, pyramidalis, rectus abdominis, and transversus abdominis muscles. In particular, the stress is felt through the
lower section of your abs.

Position
Lie back on the end of a flat bench as if performing a bench press
movement. Instead of reaching for the bar, grasp the uprights just
below the rests for the bar. Your head should be about 6 inches
from the uprights. Extend your legs straight out in front of you so
that they are parallel to the floor.

Movement Performance
As if rolling up into a ball, draw your knees up toward the
uprights while simultaneously rolling upward and back with your
hips following your knees. At the point of tightest contraction,
hold for a split second and then reverse the direction and slowly
return to the starting point. Repeat the sequence for the desired
rep count.

Hanging Leg Raise

Muscles Involved
Hanging Leg Raises stress the entire abdominal area, including the obliquus externus abdominis, obliquus internus abdominis, pyramidalis, rectus abdominis, and transversus abdominis muscles. In particular, the lower sections of the rectus abdominis are isolated.

Position
Standing on a stool or by jumping up, grasp a chinning bar with a delt-width overgrip. Hang your body straight down from the bar.

Movement Performance
Pull your knees up toward your chest as far as possible with your legs fully bent. Hold this top position for a second, then lower yourself back to the starting point and repeat for the desired number of reps.

Tips
The use of lifting straps may be helpful here due to the need to maintain your grip

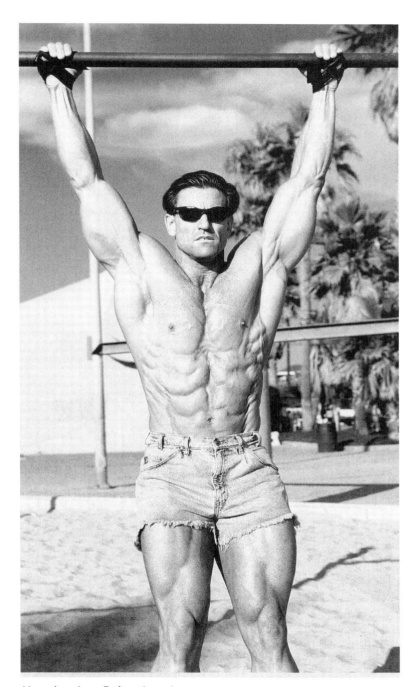

Hanging Leg Raise Lee Apperson

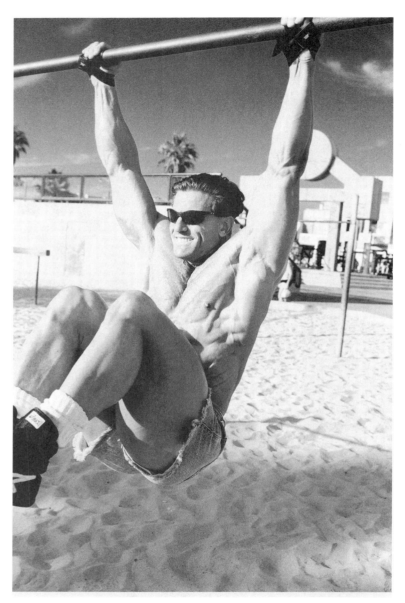

Hanging Leg Raise Lee Apperson

while supporting your entire body weight. The straps also will prevent your grip from giving out.

Additional work is forced onto your intercostals by twisting from side to side on successive reps.

Dipping Bar Leg Raise

Muscles Involved
Dipping Bar Leg Raises work the obliquus externus abdominis, obliquus internus abdominis, pyramidalis, rectus abdominis, and transversus abdominis muscles. In particular, the lower sections of the rectus abdominis are isolated.

Position
With a stool or the foot platforms provided, step up and place your back against the vertical pad. Rest your forearms on the horizontal pads while grabbing the hand grips. Allow your legs to hang straight down underneath your hips.

Movement Performance
Pull your knees up towards your chest as far as possible with your legs fully bent. Hold this top position for a second, then lower

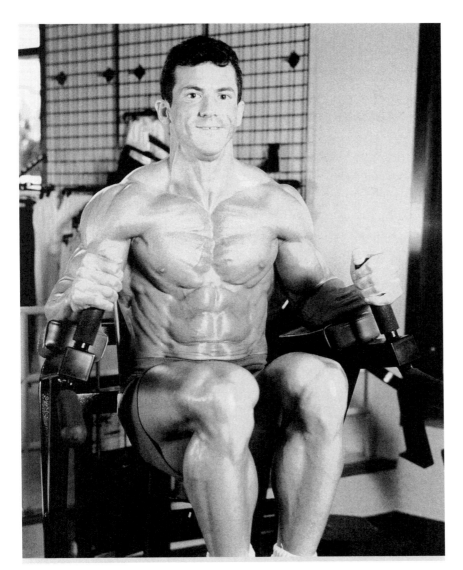

Dipping Bar Leg Raise B. J. Quinn

yourself back to the starting point and repeat for the correct repetition count.

Tips
Additional stress can be thrust onto your intercostals by twisting at the hips while drawing the knees to the opposite shoulder in an

alternating pattern of repetitions. If your legs are strong in the hip flexor area, then try some reps with them held straight out in front of you as in Leg Raises.

Side Twist with Pole

Muscles Involved
This movement is for the obliquus externus abdominis, obliquus internus abdominis, and transversus abdominis muscles. It is not true that doing thousands of them will spot trim the sides of your waist.

Note: Do not perform Side Twists if you have any lower back injury or weakness.

Position
Stand erect with your feet set slightly wider than shoulder width. Place a stretching stick across your shoulders and behind your head. Wrap your forearms over and across the stick. Be careful not to move your hips and legs during this exercise or you will lose most of the desired effect. Twists may also be performed while seated at the end of an exercise bench.

Movement Performance
Twist as far as you can to the left and right in a moderately slow rhythm for equal reps per side.

Side Bend with Cable Pulley

Muscles Involved
This movement is for the obliquus externus abdominis, obliquus internus abdominis, and transversus abdominis muscles.

Position
Attach a handle to a pulley above your head. Position yourself so that your right shoulder is underneath the handle. Stand erect

with your feet set just slightly wider than shoulder width. With your left hand, reach up and behind your head to grab the handle. In the erect starting position, the handle should be pulling against the resistance of the weight stack.

Movement Performance

Contract your left abdominal area and draw your left elbow down towards your left hip. Your shoulder will only move a few inches. Travel back and forth with a full contraction. Repeat this short range of motion for the desired rep count. Reverse your position and repeat for the right side. Be sure to train with equal reps to each side.

Tips

Do not perform this exercise if you are already thick waisted because this movement can add thickness to your waist. Additionally, only a few sets (two to three) are required for stimulation. One-arm side bends may also be performed using dumbbells.

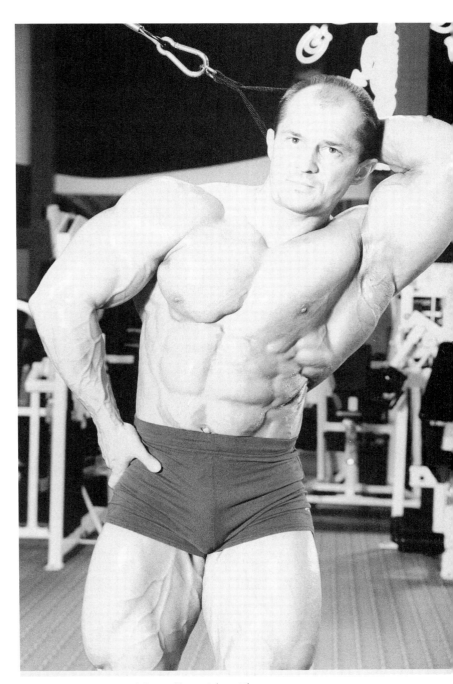

Side Bend with Cable Pulley Oleg Zhur

INDEX